FITNESS
AND WELLNESS
STRATEGIES

second edition

FITNESS AND WELLNESS STRATEGIES

Lon Seiger
Texas A&M University–Corpus Christi

Debbie Kanipe
Texas A&M University–Corpus Christi

Ken Vanderpool
Delta State University

Duke Barnes
Delta State University

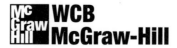

WCB McGraw-Hill

Boston, Massachusetts   Burr Ridge, Illinois   Dubuque, Iowa
Madison, Wisconsin   New York, New York   San Francisco, California   St. Louis, Missouri

WCB/McGraw-Hill

A Division of The McGraw-Hill Companies

FITNESS AND WELLNESS STRATEGIES SECOND EDITION

Recycled/acid free paper

✪ This book is printed on recycled, acid-free paper containing 10% postconsumer waste.

1 2 3 4 5 6 7 8 9 0 QPD/QPD 0 9 8 7

ISBN: 0-697-29579-6

Publisher: *Ed Bartell*
Executive editor: *Vicki Malinee*
Developmental editor: *Patricia A. Schissel*
Marketing manager: *Pamela S. Cooper*
Project manager: *Marilyn M. Sulzer*
Production supervisor: *Sandy Ludovissy*
Cover design: *Elise Lansdon*
Cover image: *© Brian Bailey/Tony Stone Images*
Photo research coordinator: *Lori Hancock*
Art editor: *Joyce Watters*
Compositor: *Shepherd, Inc.*
Typeface: *10/12 Times Roman*
Printer: *Quebecor, Inc.*

http://www.mhcollege.com

DEDICATION

To my dad for his love, support, wisdom, and, above all, strength—especially since the time of our greatest loss with mom

   —Lon Seiger

To my wife, Lucia, for her love, support, and understanding

   —Ken Vanderpool

To my parents, Barbara and Keith, for believing in me; and to my Grand Master, Sin Il Choi, for his dedicated teaching

   —Debbie Kanipe

To Linda, Chris, and Mary Elizabeth for their patience; to Robert Earl and Kitty for their support; and to Gene for his inspiration

   —Duke Barnes

Contents

PREFACE

Many people view their health as an invisible crown on their head; the only time they appreciate their health is when they have lost it to illness, disease, or injury. More than likely, these people take their health for granted and have a reactive or treatment mind-set. The authors, on the other hand, hope that you consistently appreciate your health by having a proactive or preventive philosophy! The second edition of *Fitness and Wellness Strategies* is a text designed to excite, educate, and motivate you to adopt strategies for a healthy lifestyle. When you are well, there are so many benefits, including: you feel good about yourself, you have more vitality, and you can accomplish all of your life goals.

Fitness and Wellness Strategies begins with the components of wellness and the importance of adopting healthy behaviors, including exercise. This book examines strategies to change health and fitness behaviors and to plan exercise effectively. Also, the book contains strategies to develop the health-related fitness components of cardiorespiratory endurance, strength and muscular endurance, flexibility, and body composition. Other important strategies found in the text are how to be a safe exerciser, how to stay motivated to exercise, and how to be a wise health and fitness consumer. Finally, this book provides strategies on how to eat nutritiously, how to manage your weight and fat for a lifetime, and how to cope with and manage stress.

We believe you will enjoy reading *Fitness and Wellness Strategies* and find the information important and useful. Each day of our lives we have conscious health choices to make. These choices have a cumulative effect and, over time, will either enhance or detract from our present state of well-being. The target goal for this text is for you to choose and maintain behaviors that lead to a lifestyle of fitness and wellness. Since life is a journey, let's fully enjoy the ride. One way to do this is to value our health by taking positive action for it!

TEXT FEATURES

- A **one-liner** at the beginning summarizes the **main theme** of each chapter.
- **Learning Objectives** allow you to focus on the **main goals** of each chapter.
- **Lifestyle Questions** allow you to **"buy in" or bond** to the content of each chapter.
- The material is presented in a **practical, reader-friendly style** that is **clear** and **concise.**
- Throughout each chapter, **main concepts are boldfaced** to allow you to focus on the important ideas.
- **Key terms are boldfaced** and their **definitions** follow.
- **Cartoons** can be found throughout the book to highlight the importance of humor for well-being.
- The **figures** help complement the main ideas of the text.
- The **tables** offer easy-to-follow strategies to improve health.
- **Summaries** are offered to highlight the essential information.
- **Experiential activities** are found at the end of each chapter.
- These "hands-on" learning activities bridge the gap between knowledge and application.

ANCILLARIES

As a supplement to this book, McGraw-Hill offers the following instructor and student aids:

- Instructor's Manual/Test Item File
- MicroTest III Computerized Testing Software
- WCB/McGraw-Hill Fitness and Wellness Transparency Set
- Fit Solve II aids students in assessing fitness levels, interpreting fitness testing results, and planning fitness programs.

ACKNOWLEDGMENTS

The authors wish to extend their thanks and appreciation to the contributing authors of this text: Wynn Gillan (Southeastern Louisiana University) for writing chapter 3, "Strategies to Change Health and Fitness Behavior," and Jim Hesson and Jim Hess (Black Hills State University) for writing chapter 10, "Strategies to Stay Motivated to Exercise." The authors want to especially thank Jim Hesson for his valuable suggestions to improve the overall content of this book.

The authors also want to thank John Stalmach, Publications Director at Texas A & M University–Corpus Christi for his photographic support; David Baker, Rick Milam, Bill Powell, and Robert Brown for their excellent photography; Erin Moore, Leigh Trcka, and Dr. Sarah Jordan as nutrition consultants; Lucia Vanderpool for her computerized figures; Jill Pankey and Walter Hodge for their artistic drawings; Darryl Adams, Norma Aguirre, Leslie Antici, Matt Baity, Kylie Bauder, Kerri Brown, Tracy Boyles, Danny Cohea, Rick Collier, Rosie Canales, Michael Garcia, Debbie Grossman, Kim Harwood, Tina Hernandez, Eddie Hesseltine, J. J. Jones, Jenny Kennamar, Laurita Koll, Francis Leach, Deborah Ingram, Jeff Long, Huyen-Trang Thi Mai, Michael Martinez, Angel Matthews, Audra McClain, Elaine Mora, Cindy Houston Parker, Tomeka Pennington, Margo Perez, Lance Pogue, Mark Rayburn, D'Nese Rios, Devin Sonnier, and Dewyantit Wesley for their time and patience as models; Karen Gootjes for her assistance in preparing the manuscript; and Dr. Robert Pankey, Dr. Robert Cox, Dr. Tito Guerrero III, and Dr. Robert Furgason for their administrative support.

The authors also wish to thank the following reviewers whose feedback was important to the writing of this text.

Cynthia L Pemberton
University of Missouri–Kansas City

W. Dianne Hall
University of South Florida

Ronnie Carda
University of Wisconsin–Madison

Jerry J. Wright
Pennsylvania State University at Altoona

Thomas Battinelli
Fitchburg State College

Joan Jilka
Colby Community College

1

INTRODUCTION TO FITNESS AND WELLNESS

1

WELLNESS THROUGH HEALTHY LIFESTYLES AND FITNESS

A healthy lifestyle can add life to your years and years to your life.

LEARNING OBJECTIVES

- Define health and wellness.
- Discuss the six major health and wellness components.
- Explain the wellness-illness continuum.

- Identify the six major influences on health and wellness.
- Discuss the benefits of a healthy lifestyle.
- Describe the importance of physical fitness and activity to wellness.

- Describe several strategies to achieve well-being.
- Explain the relationship of prevention to wellness.

LIFESTYLE QUESTIONS

- Are you excited about your health or do you generally take it for granted?
- How much is your health worth? Can you purchase it?
- Are the majority of health choices you now make enhancing or taking away from your well-being?

- Do you think the health choices you make today will influence your health tomorrow?
- How would you rate your desire to be healthy: strong, moderate, or weak?

INTRODUCTION

A seriously ill man went to the finest specialist in the country. After the examination, the physician presented the man with a bill for $500.

"I can't pay this, Doc. I haven't got two nickels to my name."

"If you haven't got any money," the doctor says, "why did you come to the finest specialist in the country?"

"Listen," the patient replied, "when it comes to my health, money is no object."

—Henny Youngman, comedian

Your answers in the Lifestyle Questions section will provide insight into your commitment to a healthy lifestyle. Every day we make choices that can either enhance (exercise, healthy diet) or detract (smoking, driving fast) from our present state of well-being. Although everyone desires a healthy, quality life, not everyone is willing to make the lifestyle changes necessary to bring about health improvement. However, you may be among the growing number of individuals who are striving for this richer style of life. This growth can be attributed to research findings that indicate positive lifestyle behaviors can have a significant influence on our health, quality of life, and well-being.

Wherever your health status is now, a choice of pathways lies before you. Many different paths can guide you toward better health and a richer, quality life, but only *you* can choose which trail to take, and at what speed you will travel. Choose wisely, and enjoy your journey.

HEALTH AND WELLNESS

Health is a multifaceted, dynamic quality that describes how well you are able to function at any particular point in time. Being healthy is much more than not being sick. Your health is made up of psychological, spiritual, physical, social, vocational, and environmental resources that allow you to live a satisfying and productive life. Optimal health indicates a high level of functioning and is often characterized by vitality, a zest for life, and a sense of harmony with nature and humanity.

Health is a constantly changing quality in our lives. Our health can be different from day to day and week to week due to changes in our minds, bodies, values, attitudes, beliefs, habits, and behaviors. One example of how our health can change relates to Janie, a healthy, active college sophomore. Her uncertainty about what major to declare led to excessive worrying and, eventually, to a preulcer condition. Once Janie declared a major in her junior year, she stopped worrying, her health improved, and she was better able to live her life to the fullest.

Wellness is a popular term referring to optimal health. Wellness includes an enjoyable and positive approach to a lifestyle that promotes a high level of well-being. It is a conscious commitment to growth and improvement in all areas of your life. The focus is on self-responsibility, self-fulfillment, and a richer quality of life. The wellness concept is based on the premise that adopting health-enhancing behaviors will help reduce potential disease risk factors and promote well-being. Table 1.1 highlights the benefits of achieving optimal health.

Health and wellness are closely related. Here is an example of how closely they work together: Having a disease (illness) is like a person walking backward; not being sick but not being well (neutral) is like a person standing still; and being generally healthy is like a person walking forward. When all your behaviors are health-enhancing, you are walking briskly toward optimal health (wellness).

Most Americans tend to be in neutral, neither sick nor healthy. The wellness-illness continuum (see figure 1.1) shows that wellness, or optimal health, is the highest level of functioning possible. The other end of the continuum represents the complete loss of functioning, or death. Where are you now? Place a dot where you stand on the continuum today. Place

TABLE 1.1
Major Benefits of Achieving Optimal Health

1. More "life to your years" (richer quality)
2. More "years to your life" (increased longevity)
3. A healthier mind, body, and spirit
4. Increased self-esteem and confidence
5. Greater zest for life with higher energy levels
6. More humor (fun and playfulness)
7. A positive attitude
8. Less risk for major diseases
9. Stronger immune system to ward off infections
10. More self-control and less reliance on others
11. Lower health-care costs
12. Stronger relationships
13. Improved environmental sensitivity
14. More enjoyment of your roles in life (as student, employee, etc.)
15. Better possibility of achieving your full potential in life
16. Better able to enjoy life's "moments" and experiences

FIGURE 1.1
The Wellness-Illness Continuum

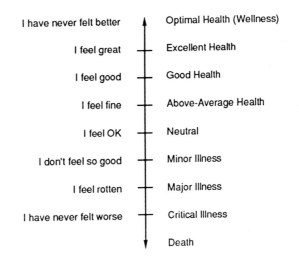

FIGURE 1.2

Health and Wellness Components

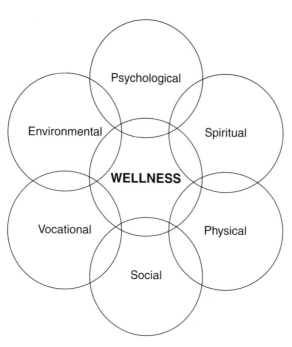

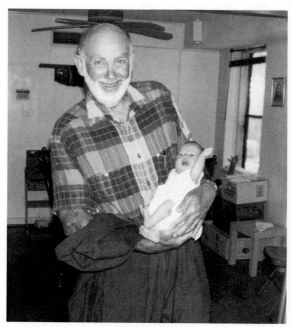

Happiness is a welcome emotion.

another dot on the continuum where you were five years ago. Which direction is your lifestyle taking you? Are your choices leading you toward a healthier and more abundant life?

HEALTH AND WELLNESS COMPONENTS

To enjoy a healthy lifestyle, many wellness components must work closely together.   Your position on the wellness-illness continuum depends largely on the daily health choices you make. It is influenced by your degree of health in each of the following wellness components: psychological, spiritual, physical, social, vocational, and environmental. The achievement of optimal health is related to being well in each of the six dimensions shown in figure 1.2.

Psychological
Psychological well-being combines both your emotional and mental states. It is not a static condition but a dynamic process that can change from day to day.

We all have our good days, our bad days, and our okay days. No one has total control over their emotional states (joy, sadness, fear, anger, shyness, loneliness, and guilt). However, emotionally healthy people strive to maintain psychological balance and know when to express their emotions appropriately and comfortably. They are also capable of showing

respect and affection for others. In the event of emotional instability, they are willing to join a support group and/or to seek professional help.

If you have mental well-being, you can embrace reality for what it is, respond positively to life's changes, and utilize healthy coping skills to deal with stress and personal problems. Also, you believe in lifelong learning. To fulfill your intellectual needs, you keep your mind active and curious, striving to learn from all of life's experiences.

Spiritual
Spiritual well-being is a positive sense of whatever provides meaning and purpose in your life. You can use your religion, philosophy, beliefs, values, faith, creed, principles, morals, or ethics to describe it. Knowing your purpose in life and being more comfortable expressing love, joy, peace, and fulfillment are part of spiritual well-being, which also includes helping yourself and others to achieve maximum potential.

Spiritual health also fosters a feeling of being connected with your inner self, significant others, and the universe. Finally, your spirituality includes having hope after setbacks and an appreciation of nature.

Physical
Physical well-being includes being physically fit, eating nutritiously, and getting adequate rest and sleep. Sexual behavior and drug and alcohol use are important to this wellness component. Physical wellness includes a personal awareness and care of the physical self, which involves regular self-tests, checkups, in-

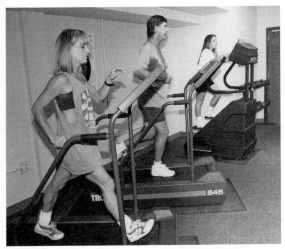

Exercising is an important component of physical well-being.

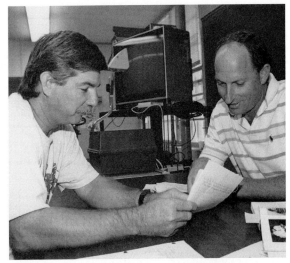

Learning at any age can be stimulating, challenging, and rewarding.

jury and disease rehabilitation, proper use of medications, and taking the appropriate steps when illness does occur.

Social

Social well-being means having satisfying, trusting relationships and interacting well with others. It includes exhibiting fairness, justice, and concern toward and appreciation of the differences in all people. The idea of being well socially suggests having a network of family members, friends, and others who can be called upon during times of need. A socially well person also feels "connected" with his or her community.

Vocational

Vocational well-being is finding meaning in and satisfaction with your school, job, and leisure pursuits. Ask yourself if what you are doing right now in life is stimulating, challenging, and rewarding. If it is, you have a high level of vocational well-being. If it is not, you may want to consider making a change and seeking further training in an area of personal interest. Last, the vocational component includes working in harmony with others to accomplish goals.

Environmental

Human survival depends on air, water, and land resources. Environmental well-being refers to the impact that this natural world has on your health. It includes protecting yourself from hazards such as secondhand smoke, which is an example of air pollution that can seriously affect your health. This component also includes being environmentally sensitive—working to preserve Earth through the four Rs: reducing, reusing, recycling, responsibility.

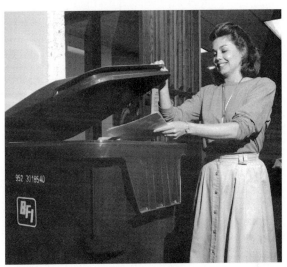

Recycling is part of being environmentally sensitive.

IMPORTANCE OF LIFESTYLE TO WELLNESS

Your lifestyle (the way you live your life) plays a key role in wellness. Your health habits are the core of your lifestyle. The health choices you make will lead toward health or illness. The effects of these daily decisions are compounded over time—day by day, week by week, month by month, and year by year. The accumulation of positive choices can lead you toward optimal health and a quality life. The accumulation of negative choices can lead you toward suffering, disease, and premature death.

Other major influences besides lifestyle influence our health. These are genetics, disease/dysfunction,

FIGURE 1.3

FIGURE 1.3

Major Influences on Wellness

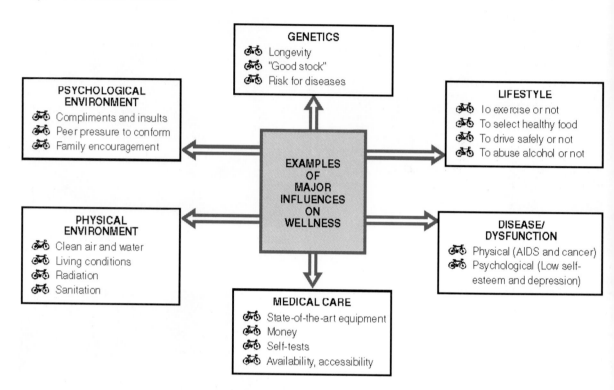

access to medical care, physical environment, and psychosocial environment. Though all are critical to wellness, most health experts rank lifestyle as the most significant factor that you have control over. Figure 1.3 provides examples of the major influences on wellness.

An unhealthy lifestyle can lead to premature death. The health problems in the United States today are quite different from those in the early 1900s. Back then, the leading causes of death were infectious diseases such as pneumonia, influenza, and tuberculosis. In America today, most of the leading causes of death are related to lifestyle (e.g., inactivity; diets high in fat, cholesterol, and calories; and smoking). Strategies for preventing and reducing the risk of dying from the leading causes of death are presented in the next section.

Many people begin living a healthy lifestyle only after they have been diagnosed with a disease (cancer, heart disease, diabetes). Fortunately, many of these individuals are able to reverse their illness and restore their health by engaging in the positive lifestyle behavior changes ordered by their physician. Unfortunately, for many others, the damage within the body may be irreversible, leading to premature death.

PREVENTING THE LEADING CAUSES OF DEATH

Many people believe that diseases and accidents—the leading causes of death in the United States—won't happen to them. Having this belief may place these individuals at an even higher risk from America's top eleven killers. Of course, the truth is that the leading causes of death don't just strike others, they strike everyone—regardless of age, sex, and race. One important key to living a richer, longer life is to reduce the risk factors that lead to life-threatening diseases and accidents.

The goal of this section is to pinpoint strategies that will lower your risk from the major killers of our time. Adopt these strategies to stack the odds in your favor for a life with more joy and self-fulfillment (wellness), and less pain and suffering (illness).

Heart Disease

Major Controllable Risk Factors
High cholesterol levels, smoking, high blood pressure, physical inactivity

Strategies to Prevent Heart Disease

1. Ask for a complete lipid (fat) profile that includes cholesterol levels. Check with your physician if levels are abnormal.
2. Follow a diet low in cholesterol, fats, and saturated fats and high in fiber, fruits, and vegetables.
3. Abstain from using tobacco.
4. Check your blood pressure regularly. If high, check with your physician to maintain levels in the desirable range.
5. Be active and engage in a regular physical fitness program.
6. Maintain levels of healthy weight and body fat.

Cancer

Major Controllable Risk Factors
Tobacco, ultraviolet radiation, diet

Secondary Risk Factors
Obesity, excessive X rays, high levels of estrogen, harmful chemicals (usually work-related), such as asbestos

Strategies to Prevent Cancer

1. Abstain from tobacco use.
2. Eat a diet high in fiber, grains, fruits, vegetables, low in fat, saturated fat, and cholesterol.
3. Protect your skin from ultraviolet radiation.
4. Maintain desirable weight and body fat levels.

Strokes

Major Controllable Stroke Risk Factors
High blood pressure, heart disease, cigarette smoking, high red blood cell count, transient ischemic attacks (small strokes)

Secondary Risk Factors for Strokes
Elevated blood cholesterol and lipids, excessive alcohol intake, physical inactivity, obesity, and taking oral contraceptives when combined with smoking

Strategies to Prevent Strokes

1. Eat a diet high in fiber, grains, fruits, vegetables, low in fat, saturated fat, and cholesterol.
2. Abstain from tobacco use.
3. Exercise regularly.
4. Keep blood pressure within normal limits.

Obstructive Pulmonary Disease (OPD)

Major Controllable Risk Factors
Smoking, air pollution

Strategies to Prevent OPD

1. Abstain from smoking tobacco.
2. Stay away from air pollution, including second-hand smoke.

Accidents

Selected Controllable Risk Factors
Drinking and driving, driving unsafely, not wearing safety belts

Strategies for Preventing Accidents

1. Always drive responsibly, defensively, and safely.
2. Do not drink and drive.
3. Do not drive with someone who is intoxicated.
4. Always wear a safety belt when riding in a motor vehicle.

Pneumonia/Influenza

Cause of Pneumonia
Bacteria, viruses (including the flu), and foreign matter (smoke) in the lungs

Strategies to Prevent Pneumonia
Receiving a vaccine is recommended for those who have previously experienced pneumonia, those with weakened immune systems, and anyone over age 50. The vaccine significantly reduces the risk of pneumonia—especially in women and others with unhealthy immune systems.

Strategies to Treat Pneumonia
Because pneumonia is so life-threatening, it is vital to see a physician immediately if you believe you have it. Symptoms include cough, a fever of 102° F or higher, shortness of breath or difficulty breathing, chills, and excessive yellow-green phlegm. Antibiotics can control bacterial pneumonia.

Cause of Influenza
Many flu viruses including Influenza A and Influenza B; transmitted by coughs, sneezes, laughs, and through conversation

Strategies to Prevent Influenza

1. Live a healthy lifestyle.
2. Do not share food or drinks.
3. Wash your hands frequently with warm water and soap.
4. Stay away from sneezers and coughers.

Strategies to Treat Influenza

Antiviral drugs can reduce the duration and severity of the flu if taken within two to three days of developing symptoms. Symptoms include fever, headache, general aches and pains, weakness, fatigue, stuffy nose, sneezing, sore throat, chest discomfort, and coughing.

Diabetes

Controllable Risk Factors

Overfatness, diet

Strategies to Prevent and Control Diabetes

1. Maintain a healthy diet.
2. Maintain a regular physical fitness program.
3. If needed, take medicine.
4. Maintain desirable weight and body fat levels.

HIV Infection/AIDS

Controllable Risk Factors

Unprotected sex, infected HIV needles, infected blood, mother-to-child

Strategies to Prevent HIV infection and AIDS

1. Maintain abstinence.
2. If sexually active, maintain a monogamous relationship with HIV-free partner, and use a double barrier including latex condoms with a spermicide.
3. Do not use IV drugs.
4. Donate own blood before surgery.
5. Both partners should take an AIDS antibody test before attempting to conceive a child.

Suicide

Controllable Risk Factors

Hopelessness, helplessness, previous suicide attempts, giving away of treasured items

Strategies to Overcome Depression and Suicidal Thoughts

1. Admit you're not well.
2. Seek help from family, friends, clergy, teachers, and professionals.
3. If needed, take medication.
4. Hang in there and don't ever give up—things will get better.

Chronic Liver Disease and Cirrhosis

Controllable Risk Factor

Consuming excessive alcohol over time

Strategies to Prevent Chronic Liver Disease and Cirrhosis

1. Abstain from alcohol.
2. If you do drink alcohol, do so only in moderation.

Homicide

Controllable Risk Factors

Anger, alcohol, hanging out in bars, guns at residence or on person, walking alone at night

Strategies to Prevent Homicide

1. Enroll in a self-defense course.
2. Control your own anger.
3. Be aware of what is going on around you at all times.
4. Project a confident, vigilant demeanor to deter potential attackers.
5. Respond to potentially hostile situations by immediately retreating or attempting to de-escalate the situation; physical confrontation should only be considered as a last resort for defending yourself.
6. When confronted by an angry, hostile individual, use the following strategies to defuse the situation:
   a. Remain calm.
   b. Maintain eye contact.
   c. Refrain from arguing.
   d. Minimize movements/gesturing.
   e. Listen.
   f. Acknowledge the person's feelings.
   g. Find solutions.
7. If you are physically attacked and the assailant is unarmed, resisting by screaming, running away, or fighting back will increase your chance of escape to 85 percent.
8. If you are physically attacked and the assailant has a weapon, do not risk your life by resisting unless you feel death is inevitable.
9. Adhere to basic safety rules:
   a. Do not answer knock on door unless you are certain who is there.
   b. Avoid walking alone, especially at night.
   c. Park in well-lit areas.
   d. Lock car doors at all times to prevent carjacking.
   e. If your vehicle breaks down, raise hood, wait inside vehicle, and ask stopping motorist to phone relative or police.

THE YEAR 2000 NATIONAL HEALTH OBJECTIVES

In 1990 the health goals of the nation were outlined in the report "Healthy People 2000." From this report,

TABLE 1.2

Healthy People 2000: Selected Objectives of the Nation

1. Reduce overweight to a prevalence of no more than 20 percent among people aged 20 and older.

2. Reduce dietary-fat intake to an average of 30 percent or less of calories and average saturated-fat intake to less than 10 percent of calories.

3. Increase complex-carbohydrate and fiber-containing foods in the diets of adults to 5 or more daily servings for vegetables (including legumes) and fruits and 6 or more daily servings for grain products.

4. Reduce alcohol consumption by people aged 14 and older to an annual average of no more than 2 gallons per person (2.5 gallons previously).

5. Reduce to no more than 30 percent the proportion of all pregnancies that are not planned. (Since 1988, an estimated 56 percent of pregnancies were unintended, unwanted, or earlier than desired.)

6. Reduce coronary heart disease deaths to no more than 100 per 100,000 (now over 135 per 100,000).

7. Reduce the prevalence of mental disorders (exclusive of substance abuse) among adults to less than 10.7 percent (now over 12 percent).

8. Reduce homicides to no more than 7.2 percent per 100,000 (now over 8.5 percent per 100,000).

9. Reduce deaths from work-related injuries to no more than 4 per 100,000 (now more than 6 per 100,000).

10. Reverse the rise in cancer deaths to achieve a rate of no more than 130 per 100,000 (now over 133 per 100,000).

11. Reduce rape and attempted rape of women aged 12–34 to no more than 225 per 100,000 (now in excess of 400 per 100,000).

12. Increase to at least 30 percent the proportion of people aged 6 and older who engage regularly, preferably daily, in light-to-moderate physical activity for at least 30 minutes per day. (Only 22 percent of people aged 18 and older are active 30 minutes or more 5 days per week; only 12 percent are active 7 days per week.)

13. Increase to at least 20 percent the proportion of people aged 18 and older who engage in vigorous physical activity that promotes the development of cardiorespiratory fitness (now about 12 percent).

14. Reduce the proportion of college students engaging in bouts of heavy drinking of alcoholic beverages to no more than 32 percent (now over 42 percent).

15. Increase to at least 50 percent the proportion of adults with high blood pressure whose blood pressure is under control (now an estimated 26 percent for those aged 18 and older).

16. Reduce the mean serum cholesterol among adults to no more than 200 mg/dl (now over 215 mg/dl).

17. Increase to at least 20 percent the proportion of people aged 18 and older who seek professional help in coping with personal and emotional problems (now slightly over 13%).

18. Increase to at least 60 percent the use of a condom at last sexual intercourse among sexually active, unmarried women aged 15–19 (now approximately 30 percent).

---

three general goals for the health of Americans were highlighted: (1) increase the span of healthy life, (2) reduce health disparities among Americans, and (3) make preventive services accessible to all Americans (see table 1.2 for selected objectives from this report).

A report card to determine progress has recently been developed for the objectives. The evaluators found that although Americans are heading in the right direction on many of the objectives, they are clearly off track in achieving others. Objectives scoring well include: more people exercising regularly and on lower-fat diets; fewer heart disease, cancer, and stroke deaths; better control of high blood pressure and cholesterol levels; and increased screening for breast and cervical cancer. The objective "fewer people overweight" was one found to be headed in the wrong direction, with one-third of Americans overweight. The report card indicated that instead of fewer Americans being overweight, more Americans than ever before are now overweight.

STRATEGIES FOR WELL-BEING

To achieve a healthy lifestyle, consider these eight important strategies.

Be Accountable

No one else is as responsible for your health as you are—not your physician, parents, friends, or partner.

If you agree that health choices are mostly within your control, you will be more apt to initiate positive lifestyle changes.

Keep a Positive Attitude

An important strategy for well-being is to keep a positive attitude toward yourself, your health, and life in general. When you keep life positive, life has a way of keeping you positive. The following piece of prose by Charles Swindol can empower you to accept responsibility for your own attitudes throughout life:

The longer I live, the more I realize the impact of attitude on life. Attitude to me is more important than facts. It is more important than the past, than education, than money, than circumstances, than failures, than successes, than what other people think or say or do. It is more important than appearance, giftedness, or skill. . . . The remarkable thing is we have a choice every day regarding the attitude we will embrace for that day. We cannot change our past. We cannot change the fact that people will act in a certain way. We cannot change the inevitable. The only thing we can do is play on the one string we have, and that is our attitude. I am convinced that life is 10% what happens to me and 90% how I react to it. As so it is with you . . . we are in charge of our attitudes.

Make Lifestyle Changes

What good is health knowledge or having positive attitudes and values if you don't apply them to life? Knowing the importance of exercise and having good intentions to be fit are admirable. However, if you don't act on this wisdom and desire, what have you accomplished? By making positive lifestyle changes, you are more likely to enjoy a high level of wellness. Chapter 3 is devoted entirely to changing health behavior.

Strive for Balance

A moderate degree of health in the six wellness components is more desirable than being strong in some and weak in others. For example, people who abuse alcohol and drugs at nightly parties may have strong social ties but are also damaging their physical health. A healthy, balanced individual can enjoy all facets of life, including school, work, family, friends, socials, and leisure time.

Engage in Variety

Variety is the spice of life and well-being. Staying with the same routine, physical activities, and health foods can lead to boredom and apathy. Consequently, enjoy the variety of all that life has to offer by engag-

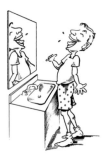

You grow up the day you have your first real laugh—at yourself.
—Ethel Barrymore

ing in many different activities. This type of lifestyle will promote fun and help prevent burnout.

Practice Moderation

Is this your belief: "Too much of a good thing is wonderful"? Any enjoyable behavior performed to excess can lead to burnout and health problems. For example, too much exercise can lead to mental fatigue and injuries. Overindulgence, even of nutritious food, can lead to excess calories and weight gain. Positive lifestyle behaviors done in moderation can keep life exciting and fun without creating unnecessary health risks. A good formula to follow is study hard, play hard, work hard—without overdoing any one!

Take Yourself and Life Lightly

Where is it written that life should always be serious and predictable? Humor (joke telling, playfulness, silliness) has been identified as the miracle drug with only funny side effects. A healthy dose of daily humor and laughter can add joy and playfulness to daily living. Physically, humor and laughter can exercise the heart muscle; improve circulation; increase alertness; and diminish tension, stress, fear, and depression. Also, a sense of humor can facilitate relationships by enhancing skills of communication.

Have It Your Way!

It's your life and your health. Since you're the owner of your mind and body, you get to make your own health decisions. You will have your own unique wellness program tailored best to meet your health needs and interests. Once you commit to the decision that your health is a top priority, you'll make everyday choices that can help prevent disease and promote well-being.

PREVENTION AND WELLNESS

An ounce of prevention is worth much more than a pound of cure. Imagine you are the owner of a prized dog. To keep her healthy, you'll want to give her the very best preventive care possible: lots of love and attention, the right amount of exercise and play, a special diet high in nutrients, the proper sleep and rest, and a positive, supportive environment. With this royal treatment, she is sure to enjoy a great, long life. Well, the same can be said for you. You also deserve the very best care so that you too can enjoy all that life has to offer. Performing at your full potential can lead to greater happiness, fulfillment, and a richer quality of life.

The time to strive for a high level of wellness is now. Why? First, the earlier that health-enhancing behaviors are adopted, the easier they are to maintain throughout life. Second, the longer a person puts off living a healthy lifestyle, the greater the risk of serious disease. For example, heart disease is America's leading cause of death. Although a heart attack may actually happen in an instant, it is decades in the making. Recent data by American Heart Association researchers clearly demonstrate that underactive children will likely become overweight, underactive adults with diseased arteries. Although adolescents may have no outward signs of **cardiovascular disease** (diseases of the heart and blood vessels), they may already show unhealthy changes in their arteries. Starting in middle age or later to live a healthy lifestyle may be too late. So, if you're ready to add *life to your years* (quality) and *years to your life* (longevity), then *let's get after it!*

SUMMARY

- Health is a multifaceted, dynamic quality that describes how well you are able to function at any particular point in time.
- Optimal health (wellness) occurs when a person fully utilizes his or her full resources. It includes an enjoyable and positive approach to a lifestyle that promotes a high level of well-being.
- Benefits of optimal health include a richer quality of life and increased longevity.
- Your wellness status, in large part, depends on your lifestyle—the daily choices you make related to your health.
- The six health and wellness components are: psychological, spiritual, physical, social, vocational, and environmental.
- Other than lifestyle, major influences on wellness include genetics, disease/dysfunction, medical care, physical environment, and psychosocial environment.
- America's top eleven killers can happen to anyone: heart disease, cancer, strokes, obstructive pulmonary disease, accidents, pneumonia/influenza, diabetes, HIV infection, suicide, chronic liver disease and cirrhosis, and homicide.
- One important key to living a richer, longer life is to adopt strategies that reduce the risk factors that lead to life-threatening diseases and accidents.
- The U.S. government is actively involved in promoting health and preventing disease by identifying the Year 2000 National Objectives, which serve as health goals for all Americans. The report card to assess progress found that though most objectives are being met, some are still off track.
- The eight strategies for well-being include: be accountable, keep a positive attitude, make lifestyle changes, strive for balance, engage in variety, practice moderation, take yourself and life lightly, and have it your way!
- An ounce of disease prevention and health promotion is worth much more than a pound of cure.
- There are two reasons why now is the time to strive for a high level of wellness. One, the earlier that health-enhancing behaviors are adopted, the easier they are to maintain throughout life. Second, the longer that a person puts off living a healthy lifestyle, the greater the risk of serious disease.

ACTIVITY   1A

HEALTH-STYLE SELF-TEST

Name _____   **To be submitted: Yes   No**

Date _____   **If yes, due date** _____

Class _____ Section _____   **Score** _____

PURPOSE
To examine your lifestyle behaviors. The seven key behaviors examined in this self-test apply to most Americans. Certain sections may not apply to individuals with certain diseases and handicaps.

DIRECTIONS
1. The Health-Style Self-Test has seven sections and can be found on the next two pages. Complete each section by circling the number that corresponds to the best answer describing the way you live.

2. Determine your score by totaling the circled numbers within each section (not all sections together).

3. Answer the questions in the Results section.

RESULTS
1. Record your scores for each of the seven sections:

   Tobacco Use _____

   Alcohol and Other Drugs _____

   Nutrition _____

   Exercise/Fitness _____

   Emotional Health _____

   Safety _____

   Disease Prevention _____

2. In which sections did you score 8 or below?

3. What three changes can you make to improve your health?

HEALTH-STYLE SELF-TEST

All of us want optimal health. But many of us do not know how to achieve it. That's what this brief test, adapted from one created by the U.S. Public Health Service, is all about. The behaviors covered in the test are recommended for most Americans. (Some of them may not apply to people with certain diseases or disabilities, or to pregnant women, who may require special advice from their physicians.) After you take the quiz, add up your score for each section.

Tobacco Use

If you never use tobacco, enter a score of 10 for this section and go to the next section.

	Almost Always	Sometimes	Never
1. I avoid using tobacco.	2	1	0
2. I smoke only low-tar-and-nicotine cigarettes, or I smoke a pipe or cigars, or I use smokeless tobacco.	2	1	0

Tobacco Score: _____

Alcohol and Other Drugs

	Almost Always	Sometimes	Never
1. I avoid alcohol, or I drink no more than 1 or 2 drinks a day.	4	1	0
2. I avoid using alcohol or other drugs as a way of handling stressful situations or problems in my life.	2	1	0
3. I am careful not to drink alcohol when taking medications, such as for colds or allergies, or when pregnant.	2	1	0
4. I read and follow the label directions when using prescribed and over-the-counter drugs.	2	1	0

Alcohol and Other Drugs Score: _____

Nutrition

	Almost Always	Sometimes	Never
1. I eat a variety of foods each day, including 5 or more servings of fresh fruits and vegetables.	3	1	0
2. I limit the amount of fat and saturated fat in my diet.	3	1	0
3. I avoid skipping meals.	2	1	0
4. I limit the amount of salt and sugar I eat.	2	1	0

Nutrition Score: _____

Exercise/Fitness

	Almost Always	Sometimes	Never
1. I engage in moderate exercise for 20 to 60 minutes, 3 to 5 times a week.	4	1	0
2. I maintain a healthy weight, avoiding overweight and underweight.	2	1	0
3. I do exercises to develop muscular strength and endurance at least twice a week.	2	1	0
4. I spend some of my leisure time participating in physical activities such as gardening, bowling, golf, or baseball.	2	1	0

Exercise/Fitness Score: _____

Emotional Health

	Almost Always	Sometimes	Never
1. I enjoy being a student and I have a job or do other work that I like.	2	1	0
2. I find it easy to relax and express my feelings freely.	2	1	0
3. I manage stress well.	2	1	0
4. I have close friends, relatives, or others I can talk to about personal matters and call on for help.	2	1	0
5. I participate in group activities (such as church and community organizations) or hobbies that I enjoy.	2	1	0

Emotional Health Score: _____

Safety

	Almost Always	Sometimes	Never
1. I wear a seat belt while riding in a car.	2	1	0
2. I avoid driving while under the influence of alcohol or other drugs.	2	1	0
3. I obey traffic rules and the speed limit when driving.	2	1	0
4. I read and follow instructions on the labels of potentially harmful products or substances, such as household cleaners, poisons, and electrical appliances.	2	1	0
5. I avoid smoking in bed.	2	1	0

Safety Score: _____

Disease Prevention

	Almost Always	Sometimes	Never
1. I know the warning signs of cancer, diabetes, heart attack, and stroke.	2	1	0
2. I avoid overexposure to the sun and use sunscreens.	2	1	0
3. I get recommended medical screening tests (such as blood pressure checks and Pap smears), immunizations, and booster shots.	2	1	0
4. I practice monthly breast/testicle self-exams.	2	1	0
5. I am not sexually active *or* I have sex with only one mutually faithful, uninfected partner *or* I always engage in "safer sex" (using condoms and a spermicide containing nonoxynol-9) *and* I do not share needles.	2	1	0

Disease Prevention Score: _____

What Your Scores Mean to You

Scores of 9 and 10

Excellent! Your answers show that you are aware of the importance of this area to your health. More important, you are putting your knowledge to work for you by practicing good health habits. As long as you continue to do so, this area should not pose a serious health risk. It's likely that you are setting an example for your family and friends to follow. Since you got a very high test score on this part of the test, you may want to consider other areas where your scores indicate room for improvement.

Scores of 6 to 8

Your health practices in this area are good, but there is room for improvement. Look again at the items you answered with a "Sometimes" or "Almost Never." What changes can you make to improve your score? Even a small change can often help you achieve better health.

Scores of 3 to 5

Your health risks are showing! Would you like more information about the risks you are facing and about why it is important for you to change these behaviors? Perhaps you need help in deciding how to successfully make the changes you desire. In either case, help is available.

Scores of 0 to 2

Obviously, you were concerned enough about your health to take the test, but your answers show that you may be taking serious and unnecessary risks with your health. Perhaps you are not aware of the risks and what to do about them. You can easily get the information and help you need to improve, if you wish. The next step is up to you.

Source: Healthstyle: A Self-Test. Office of Disease Prevention and Health Promotion. Department of Health and Human Services, Washington, DC.

A C T I V I T Y   *1B*

THE WELLNESS WHEEL

Name _____   *To be submitted:*   Yes   No

Date _____   *If yes, due date* _____

Class _____   *Section* _____   *Score* _____

PURPOSE
To assess your current level of wellness in the six dimensions.

PROCEDURES
1. Review the six wellness components found on pages 4 through 5 in chapter 1.

2. Place a dot on each line of the Wellness Wheel (found in figure 1.4) that best represents where you feel you are now. Dots placed close to the inner circle (hub) represent a lower level of health whereas dots placed near the outer circle (rim) indicate a high level of health.

3. Connect the dots.

4. Answer the questions in the Results section.

RESULTS
1. How balanced is your wellness wheel? (Will your wheel roll or crash after the first turn?)

2. Are you close to achieving a high level of health in each dimension?   Yes   No   What are your strengths? What are your weaknesses?

	Strengths	*Weaknesses*
1.	_____	_____
2.	_____	_____
3.	_____	_____
4.	_____	_____

3. What behaviors can you eliminate, modify, or adopt to improve your health?

Eliminate: _____

Modify: _____

Adopt: _____

FIGURE 1.4
The Wellness Wheel

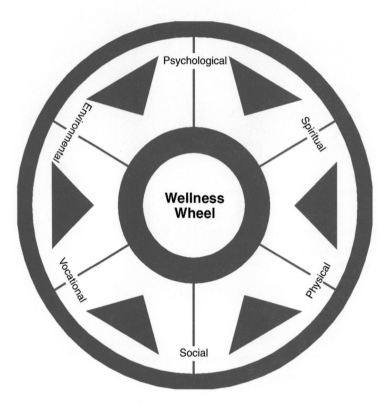

2

THE IMPORTANCE OF PHYSICAL FITNESS TO WELLNESS

"If exercise could be packed into a pill, it would be the single most widely prescribed and beneficial medicine in the nation"—*The National Institutes of Health.*

LEARNING OBJECTIVES

- Describe the importance of physical fitness and activity to wellness.

- Define physical fitness and exercise.

- Discuss the latest recommendations for being physically active.

- Explain the harmful effects of a sedentary lifestyle.

- Identify the benefits of being physically fit and active.

- Explore several of the hypokinetic diseases linked to inactivity.

- Identify and briefly describe the five components of health-related fitness.

- Identify and briefly describe the six components of skill-related fitness.

LIFESTYLE QUESTIONS

- Would you classify your lifestyle as more active or more sedentary?

- Are you currently physically fit?

- In general, does your physical activity add up to at least thirty minutes a day?

- If given a choice, would you rather be active or inactive?

- Do you actually enjoy the time during exercise and being physically active?

INTRODUCTION

To enjoy a high level of wellness, it is essential to be physically active and fit. Even moderate increases in physical activity and fitness levels will produce health and wellness benefits. When you are physically active and engaging in a regular exercise program, the various systems of your body can function more efficiently.

Exercise is defined as any human movement or physical activity. Exercise includes the full spectrum of movement—from formal activities such as calisthenics (push-ups and sit-ups) and movements performed in sports, games, and dance to informal activities such as walking, swimming, bicycling, and jogging. Exercise is the behavior that leads to physical fitness.

Physical fitness is defined as the optimal functioning of the body in all of its daily activities. A high level of physical fitness goes beyond being simply active during the day; it also includes a regular and effective exercise program. By being physically fit, you can perform your everyday tasks and still have abundant reserve energy left to meet other physical demands such as intramural and recreational sports, hobbies, and other leisure pursuits. Also, being fit allows you to have ample energy to meet most unexpected emergencies and crisis situations whenever they occur.

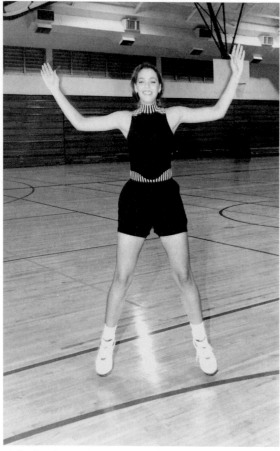 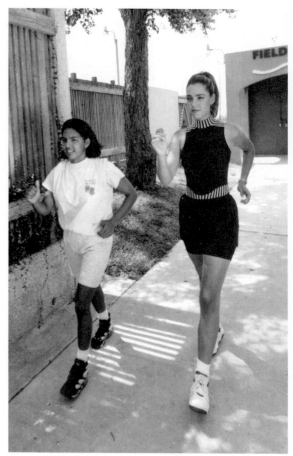

Calisthenics and walking are two popular forms of exercise.

THE LATEST RECOMMENDATIONS

The Surgeon General's Report on Physical Activity and Health recently released the following recommendations for adults and especially the large sedentary population of the United States:

1. Set a goal to accumulate at least thirty minutes or more of physical activity—time spent can be continuous or in bouts of at least ten minutes provided it totals thirty minutes per day (expending 150 calories a day through exercise will allow us to become moderately fit and pave the way to improved health and less risk for health problems associated with inactivity).
2. Exercise at moderate intensity.
3. Exercise for most, and preferably all, days of the week.
4. No particular type of activity was singled out as being more or less effective—as long as it is performed regularly and at the level of exertion that raises and sustains the metabolic rate for the total thirty minutes.

5. People who currently meet or exceed this recommended minimal standard may derive additional health and fitness benefits from being more physically active or including more vigorous activity in their daily living.

A final note from the report: A lack of time, goals, and internal motivation prevents people from being physically active, although most of the general public would admit they would feel better with regular physical activity.

The latest research into exercise is finding that even low levels of exercise can contribute to your health. Although optimal benefits from exercise can only be achieved by meeting selected criteria, any form of exercise is beneficial. Research has shown remarkable benefits through the accumulation of physical activity even in periodic, short bouts. One can gain most of the necessary health benefits through common, everyday physical activity, rather than only activities normally associated with physical fitness, like running or swimming. This would include such activities as taking the stairs instead of using an elevator or escalator, gardening and yard-

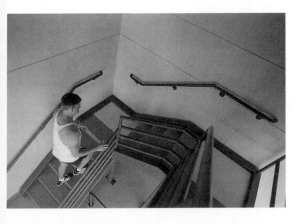

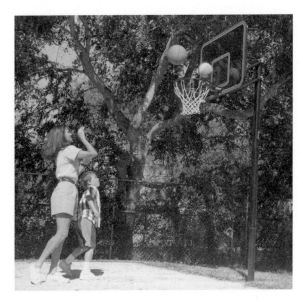

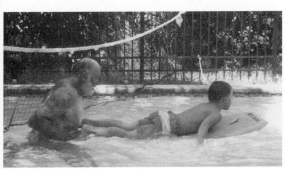

To become more active throughout your day: take the stairs, play with children, or do more physical activities.

work, housework, and playing with our children and pets. For further evidence, Stanford University researchers studied the physical activity and lifestyle characteristics of nearly 17,000 Harvard alumni. For those subjects who smoked, were hypertensive, or obese, the researchers found they still had greater life expectancy as long as they were physically active.

At one time, the motto for exercisers was "go for the burn" and "no pain, no gain." Is it any wonder so many people turned away from exercise with this prevailing attitude? The latest research now focuses less on what type of activity we do, or even for the duration of time we do it, as long as we meet our requirement of thirty minutes for most, if not all, days of the week (see fig. 2.1).

THE SEDENTARY LIFESTYLE

According to the Centers for Disease Control and Prevention, only about 15 percent of people in America are active enough to realize the health benefits of physical activity. Sixty percent of us are somewhat active, meaning we do not get the recommended amount of physical activity. This leaves 25 percent, or 1 in 4 adults, who report no exercise in their daily lives. Perhaps if more people realized how easy it is to total thirty minutes of daily activity, then

fewer people in America would be suffering the harmful effects of their sedentary lifestyle—heart disease, stroke, cancer, and diabetes. As mentioned, surveys have found that a lack of time, goals, and internal motivation prevents people from being physically active. Chapter 10 addresses strategies to counteract these barriers and stay motivated to exercise.

We are designed to move; if we sit or lie down too long, our bodies begin to feel sluggish and lazy. Before the age of technology, physical activity was essential for survival. How times have changed! Today most jobs are sedentary in nature and do not require the demanding physical exertion that was once needed. Plus, we have become a nation of spectators with television, easy access to movies and videos, and more athletic events to watch. Consequently, we have to offset the inactivity patterns of our daily routines through conscious choices to be more physically active.

To offset our electronic world that encourages a sedentary lifestyle, participate in a structured physical fitness program and choose to be active whenever possible. A structured physical fitness program will include effective and enjoyable exercises performed on a regular basis. These are exercises that are specifically chosen for their health-related benefits, such as swimming and walking to improve cardiorespiratory endurance and weight training to increase muscular strength and muscular endurance.

FIGURE 2.1

Daily Activities to Improve Health and Fitness

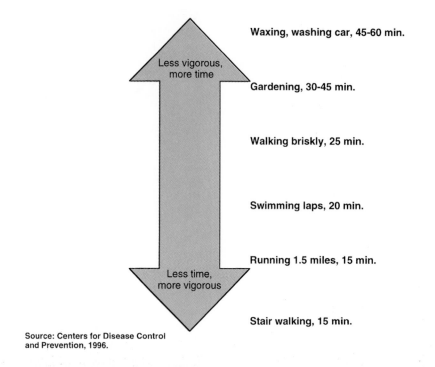

Less vigorous, more time

Less time, more vigorous

Waxing, washing car, 45-60 min.

Gardening, 30-45 min.

Walking briskly, 25 min.

Swimming laps, 20 min.

Running 1.5 miles, 15 min.

Stair walking, 15 min.

Source: Centers for Disease Control and Prevention, 1996.

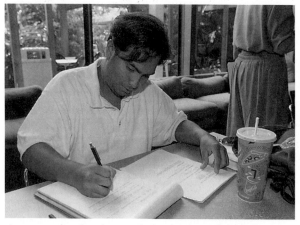

An example of sedentary behavior is studying.

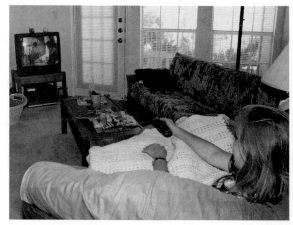

Too much inactivity can place your health at risk.

Choose to be more active! In addition to a workout program, be more active throughout the day. Walking across campus, taking the stairs, throwing a Frisbee or football to a friend, and taking short exercise breaks while studying are examples of conscious decisions to become more active and less sedentary in life.

Both a structured physical fitness program and choosing to be more active can allow you to meet your body's needs for daily exercise. "If you don't use it, you lose it" is a popular saying that directly applies to the many different systems and organs of your body. Living an active lifestyle by moving your body is an essential part of developing and maintaining a healthy lifestyle.

BENEFITS OF BEING PHYSICALLY FIT

Many health and wellness benefits are associated with being physically fit. On the other hand, many **hypokinetic diseases** or health problems are associated with a *lack* of activity or a sedentary lifestyle (see fig 2.2). In the word *hypokinetic*, "hypo" stands for "lack of" and "kinetic" stands for "energy." Hy-

FIGURE 2.2
Health Problems Linked to Inactivity

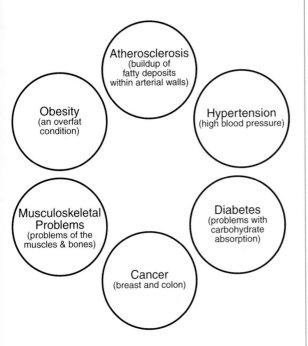

pokinetic diseases include heart disease, musculoskeletal problems, obesity, diabetes, high blood pressure, and breast and colon cancer.

Think about your lifestyle. Are you living a physically active lifestyle and enjoying the many benefits that go along with it? Or are you living a physically inactive lifestyle and increasing your chances of developing a hypokinetic disease? Some major benefits of being physically fit and leading an active lifestyle are highlighted next.

Decreased Risk for Coronary Heart Disease (CHD)

The American Heart Association has recently identified physical inactivity as one of the four primary risk factors for CHD. Therefore, if you lead a sedentary lifestyle, you have a greater likelihood of suffering a heart attack. One way exercise can decrease your risk for CHD is by lowering low-density lipoprotein (LDL), the bad cholesterol, while raising high-density lipoprotein (HDL), the good cholesterol. Although there are many other risk factors, including some that are inherited, being active and physically fit can reduce your chances of premature death from CHD.

Fewer Musculoskeletal Problems

Low back pain and pains from the neck to the feet are often associated with lack of exercise and activity. Research indicates that as many as 80 percent of us will experience lower back problems and the accompanying pain during our lives. A problem common among older adults and especially postmenopausal women is **osteoporosis**—a chronic condition in which the bones become weaker. Although musculoskeletal problems do require medical guidance, appropriate forms of physical activity are often recommended as both preventative measures and treatments. Being fit and physically active today can prevent muscle and bone problems over the years.

Increased Work Efficiency

In a pure sense, all human movement may be defined as **work** (the force required to move the body and other objects over a distance). Whether we perceive something as work or not often depends on the effort required of us. As our bodies become more physically fit, daily activity demands and choices are accomplished more efficiently. Stronger muscles are able to lift a weight (books, groceries, spare tire, barbells) with less effort. Also, activities like climbing a flight of stairs that once made our hearts race and caused shortness of breath will become easier as our body becomes more fit.

Fat Reduction

Research has consistently shown that too many Americans are **obese.** Obesity can lead to numerous health problems such as heart disease, respiratory and circulatory problems, diabetes, and breast cancer and colon cancer. The systems of the body must work harder because of the extra weight and fat. A physically active lifestyle helps to maintain a proper balance of fat tissue to lean muscle tissue.

Decreased Risk for Diabetes

Diabetes is a condition where there are problems with carbohydrate absorption. One of the leading causes of death in the United States, diabetes is associated with several other problems such as heart disease, blindness, stroke, and poor blood vessel circulation. Along with a healthy diet, exercise is an important part of managing diabetes and its related health problems.

Reduced Hypertension

Hypertension, or high blood pressure, is a problem for about 20 percent of the population. People who have mild and moderate levels of high blood pressure make up another 20 percent. African Americans and Hispanics are more likely to have high blood pressure than whites, and males are more likely to have it than females. The normal level of blood pressure is 120/80. The 120 is the systolic number, measuring the amount of pressure within the arteries when the heart contracts. The 80 is the diastolic number, measuring the amount of pressure with the arteries when the heart relaxes.

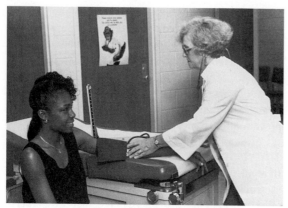

Keep your blood pressure within normal limits to prevent diseases of the heart and blood vessels.

Heart and blood vessel diseases are more common among people with high blood pressure. Exercise is one of the most effective methods for preventing high blood pressure, and treating mild and moderate cases of this dangerous health condition.

Decreased Risk for Breast Cancer and Colon Cancer

As cancer deaths continue to rise, more research has been conducted to help determine the causes of various forms of cancer. Inactive lifestyles have been linked to breast cancer and colon cancer, two leading causes of cancer-related deaths among adults. Enjoying an active lifestyle and being physically fit can reduce your risk for breast and/or colon cancer.

Fewer Problems Associated with a Heart Attack

Besides preventing heart disease, effective exercise programs are important parts of rehabilitation programs for those who survive heart attacks. In addition, people with fit bodies may have a less severe heart attack and a better chance of surviving one if it does occur.

Increased Quantity and Quality of Life

The benefits of an active and fitness-oriented lifestyle can be measured in both quantity and quality of life. Although research indicates that physically active individuals can experience a longer life, the quality of those years may be even more important. People who are physically active and fit have better resources to enjoy a richer life by reaching their full potential. Feeling good about yourself, learning to enjoy every day, and improving the quality of your life may be the ultimate benefits of a physically active lifestyle and regular exercise program.

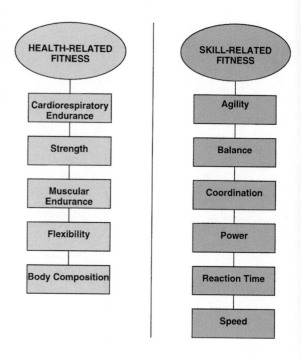

FIGURE 2.3
Components of Health-Related and Skill-Related Fitness

PHYSICAL FITNESS COMPONENTS

Physical fitness is divided into two categories: health-related fitness and skill-related fitness (see fig. 2.3). **The components of health-related fitness help promote health and prevent disease, whereas the components of skill-related fitness are more associated with better performance in games and sports.** Because of their relationship to wellness, the five health-related components should serve as the primary focus when beginning an exercise program or assessing your current level of physical fitness. Table 2.1 highlights many types of activities that can improve your fitness in the five health-related components.

Although a brief summary follows for each health-related component, a much more in-depth discussion can be found in chapters 5 to 8.

Health-Related Fitness Components

1. **Cardiorespiratory Endurance.** Cardiorespiratory endurance is described as the condition of the circulatory and respiratory systems. The level of cardiorespiratory endurance is an indication of the body's ability to transport and use oxygen. A fit person can sustain physical activity for relatively long periods of time without becoming too fatigued.

TABLE 2.1
Physical Activity and the Health-Related Components

Physical Activity	Flexibility	Cardiorespiratory Endurance	Muscular Strength and Endurance	
			Lower Body	*Upper Body*
Aerobics class	**	**	**	**
Badminton	**	**	**	
Bench-stepping		**	**	
Bicycling		**	**	
Board-sailing		**	**	**
Bowling			**	**
Calisthenics		**	**	**
Canoeing		**		**
Dance, aerobic	**	**	**	**
Gardening	**	**	**	**
Golf (no cart)	**	**	**	
Gymnastics	**	**	**	**
Hiking	**	**	**	
Ice-skating		**	**	
Kayaking	**	**		**
Martial arts	**	**	**	**
Pickle ball	**	**	**	
Push-mowing		**	**	**
Racquetball		**	**	**
Rock-climbing	**	**	**	**
Rollerblading		**	**	
Rowing		**	**	**
Running		**	**	**
Sailing	**			**
Skiing, cross-country	**	**	**	**
Skiing, downhill	**	**	**	
Stair-climbing		**	**	
Swimming	**	**	**	**
Tennis		**	**	**
Volleyball		**	**	**
Walking, fitness	**	**	**	
Weight training	**		**	**
Yoga	**		**	**

Cardiorespiratory endurance is considered to be the most important component of health-related fitness because of its value in combating heart disease, strokes, high blood pressure, obesity, and stress. Cardiorespiratory endurance is also important to many types of work, play, and sports activities.

2. **Strength.** Strength is defined as the ability of the muscles to exert a single maximum force. A fit person can perform daily activities—pushing, pulling, lifting, carrying—without strain or undue fatigue.

3. **Muscular Endurance.** Muscular endurance is the ability to repeat submaximal contractions. A fit person can repeat movements for long periods of time without undue fatigue.
4. **Flexibility.** Flexibility is defined as the range of motion in a joint. A flexible person can move the body joints through a greater range of motion.

   In past years, flexibility has been the most over-looked component of health-related fitness. Today, stretching exercises are considered an important part of any physical fitness program.
5. **Body Composition.** Body composition primarily describes the ratio of lean body weight (muscle, bone, and other tissue) to fat. A fit person will have a desirable level of body fat—not too much and not too little.

Skill-Related Fitness Components

1. **Agility.** Agility reflects our ability to change direction quickly and accurately during movement. It is a necessary skill to participate in sports and games such as tennis and basketball where there is constant stopping, starting, and changing direction.
2. **Balance.** Balance is the ability to maintain equilibrium while moving or standing still. Activities such as roller-skating, in-line skating, and gymnastics require good balance.
3. **Coordination.** Coordination indicates the ability to use senses with the body parts to perform movement tasks. It is required in all sports, especially those in which hand-eye coordination (baseball, racquetball) or foot-eye coordination (soccer, football) is required.
4. **Power.** Power is the ability to apply a force at a high rate of speed. Weight lifters need power to lift heavy weights. Football players need power to effectively block and tackle. Power is also evident when a baseball player hits a home run or a pitcher throws a fastball for a strike.
5. **Reaction time.** Reaction time is the elapsed time between a stimulus and the resulting response. Sprinters need good reaction. After hearing the horn, the quickness of the runner in getting out of the blocks will likely have some effect of the outcome of the race.
6. **Speed.** Speed deals with the rate at which a movement is performed. Speed will prove beneficial in most sports.

SUMMARY

- To enjoy a high level of wellness, it is essential to be physically active and fit.

- Exercise is defined as any human movement or physical activity and is the behavior that leads to physical fitness.
- Physical fitness is defined as the optimal functioning of the body in all of its daily activities.
- The *Surgeon General's Report on Physical Activity and Health* recently released several recommendations for adults and especially the large sedentary population of the United States.
- The latest research into exercise is finding that even low levels of exercise can contribute to your health.
- At one time, the motto for exercisers was "go for the burn" and "no pain, no gain." The latest research now focuses less on what type of activity we do, or even on the duration of time we do it, as long as we meet our requirement of thirty minutes for most, if not all, days of the week.
- According to the Centers for Disease Control and Prevention, only about 15 percent of people in America are active enough to realize the health benefits of physical activity. Sixty percent of us are somewhat active, which leaves 25 percent, or 1 in 4 adults, who report no exercise in their daily lives.
- To offset our electronic world that encourages a sedentary lifestyle, participate in a structured physical fitness program and choose to be active whenever possible.
- Many health and wellness benefits are associated with being physically fit, such as decreased risk for heart disease and increased quantity and quality of life.
- Many hypokinetic diseases or health problems are associated with a lack of activity or a sedentary lifestyle. Hypokinetic diseases include heart disease, musculoskeletal problems, obesity, diabetes, high blood pressure, and breast and colon cancer.
- Physical fitness is divided into the two categories of health-related fitness and skill-related fitness. Health-related fitness is composed of cardiorespiratory endurance, muscular strength, muscular endurance, flexibility, and body composition. Skill-related fitness is composed of agility, balance, coordination, power, reaction time, and speed.
- Because of their relationship to wellness, the five health-related components should serve as the primary focus when beginning an exercise program or assessing your current level of physical fitness.

ACTIVITY *2*

ASSESSING YOUR FITNESS AND LEISURE PATTERNS

Name _____   To be submitted: Yes   No

Date _____   If yes, due date _____

Class _____   Section _____   Score _____

PURPOSE
To determine your patterns in your fitness habits and leisure activities.

DIRECTIONS
Complete the questionnaire and then answer the questions in the Results section.

FITNESS AND LEISURE QUESTIONNAIRE

1. Which of the following leisure activities do you enjoy on a regular basis? Check all that apply.

   ☐ Playing cards   ☐ Swimming   ☐ Racquet sports
   ☐ Board games   ☐ Fishing   ☐ Snow skiing
   ☐ Video games   ☐ Camping   ☐ Water skiing
   ☐ Watching TV   ☐ Canoeing   ☐ Hiking
   ☐ Reading   ☐ Horsemanship   ☐ Climbing
   ☐ Painting   ☐ Shooting sports   ☐ Rappelling
   ☐ Sewing/Needlework   ☐ Basketball   ☐ Jet skiing
   ☐ Crafts   ☐ Volleyball   ☐ Windsurfing
   ☐ Other _____   ☐ Other _____

2. How would you describe your regular leisure activity choices?

   ☐ Sedentary   ☐ Moderately active
   ☐ Slightly active   ☐ Very active

3. Which of the following exercise activities do you enjoy on a regular basis?

   ☐ Swimming   ☐ Aerobic dance
   ☐ Biking   ☐ Step aerobics
   ☐ Walking   ☐ Water aerobics
   ☐ Jogging/Running   ☐ Stair climbing
   ☐ Flexibility exercises ☐ Other
   ☐ Skiing _____
   ☐ Rowing _____

4. How often do you exercise for fitness?

   ☐ Daily   ☐ Occasionally
   ☐ 3–6 times per week   ☐ Seldom

5. How long do you usually exercise during each workout?

☐ 15 minutes or less   ☐ 46–60 minutes

☐ 16–30 minutes   ☐ I don't exercise

☐ 31–45 minutes

RESULTS

1. From the questionnaire, what can you conclude about your leisure patterns?

2. From the questionnaire, what can you conclude about your fitness/exercise patterns?

3. Is there any relationship between your patterns of exercise and how active your patterns are for leisure time?   Yes   No   Explain.

3

STRATEGIES TO CHANGE HEALTH AND FITNESS BEHAVIOR

Changing most health behaviors does not have to be complex. Just plan well and then commit to your plan!

LEARNING OBJECTIVES

- Define the term behaviors.

- Examine what motivates behavior.

- Discuss the four major strategies for changing behavior.

- Explain the purpose of setting goals for changing behavior.

- Discuss the importance of antecedents and consequences to change.

- Explain the importance of keeping a journal to observe behavior.

- Identify six techniques to achieve your target behavior.

LIFESTYLE QUESTIONS

- What behaviors have you changed successfully?

- What behaviors have you tried to change without success?

- Is there a behavior you are currently changing?

- Is there a behavior you would like to change?

- Do you currently exercise on a regular basis?

- If you're not a regular exerciser, would you like to change your behavior to become one?

INTRODUCTION

To change something about yourself can be one of the most satisfying maturing experiences you can have. It can also be very challenging. To make a change, you have to want to, know how to, believe you can, and use a number of proven techniques. This chapter will provide you with the knowledge and skills necessary to make health and fitness changes in your life.

Buckling your safety belt, exercising, and choosing fruits and vegetables for snacks are examples of helpful habits you can adopt to improve or maintain your health. You may already engage in these or other types of healthy lifestyle patterns. It is also common, however, for us to engage in patterns that place our health at risk, such as inactivity, smoking, and abusing alcohol. The keys to well-being are to maintain our healthy behaviors while identifying and changing those that are unhealthy. Making successful changes to improve our health gives us feelings of

self-control and the confidence that we can initiate other healthy changes in our lives. For example, to begin and maintain an exercise program can lead to other successful health changes, including healthy snacking and improved anger control.

WHAT ARE BEHAVIORS?

Behaviors include both physical and cognitive responses or actions that are triggered by some type of stimuli—either internal or external. An example of a physical response would be to eat in response to anxiety. Research has shown that as anxiety levels rise, the frequency of oral behaviors such as eating increases. This type of eating is not related to sensations of hunger, but rather appears to be an unconscious response linked to one's level of anxiety.

Cognitive behaviors differ from physical behaviors. Instead of being automatic, cognitive behaviors involve specific thought patterns. These thought

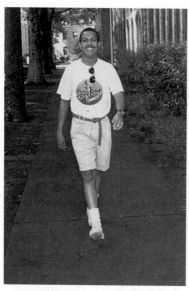

A regular exercise program is an effective method for controlling stress.

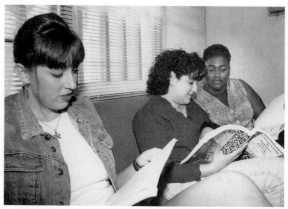

Learning new information is a motivating factor to read books.

patterns (referred to as **internal dialogue,** or **self-talk**) frequently become so ingrained that they often go unnoticed by the individual. Even though much of our own self-talk goes unnoticed, it nonetheless shapes our attitudes and colors our perception of the world around us. Fortunately, it is possible through practice to become aware of these thought patterns and to learn how to modify and control them. Here is an example of a cognitive behavior as it relates to eating and how common it is to engage in some form of internal dialogue or self-talk.

Jim was studying for a test when his roommate Bob returned with a pepperoni pizza. When Bob asked Jim if he were hungry, Jim quickly responded with a no. Bob opened the pizza box and began eating a slice. Seconds later, Jim smelled the pizza and when he looked up from his study notes, he saw the steam rising from the hot pizza. "I guess I changed my mind after all and would enjoy some pizza," said Jim.

This sudden change in Jim's level of hunger was the result of an internal dialogue that was triggered by the pizza's smell and sight. If Jim were asked what he said to himself that changed his mind, he might have replied, "When I smelled that pizza, my mouth began to water (a physical response), and I began thinking to myself how delicious a bite would taste. Then, when I saw the steam rising and observed the satisfied look on my roommate's face, I said to myself I knew I would have to have some pizza (cognitive response)."

In our lives, stimuli include events, people, places, things, and even our thoughts. Our response to a given stimulus is based on our perception of that stimulus. If our perception is a composite of our beliefs, values, habits, attitudes, emotional state, and previous life experiences, it follows that the same stimulus may trigger a wide range of responses among various individuals. For example, to relieve anxiety, you may choose to exercise while your friends may choose to eat. Everyone responds differently to stimuli. Identifying our thoughts, feelings, and the actions that lead to our reaction to stimuli is an important first step in understanding why we behave the way we do.

WHAT MOTIVATES BEHAVIOR?

What factors in life motivate us? What gets us out of bed in the morning? What motivates us to attend school, get a job, or read this book? In most cases, our goals, personal values, beliefs, knowledge, attitudes, and unmet needs drive us. And often we are motivated by other individuals—we want to behave in ways we feel are expected of us.

You perform specific behaviors to seek pleasure or avoid pain. When you want something badly enough, it will be the depth of your desire that will determine the strength of your motivation. For example, if you have a strong desire to begin and maintain an exercise program, your motivation will be higher to be successful. The reverse is also true.

Once you have reached the goal that motivated you, the original goal loses its power to drive you. To regain motivation, you must set another goal. For example, let's say you set a goal to begin a swimming program. You start exercising and have reached your original goal. Now, to stay motivated, you must set a new goal to maintain your swimming program.

Goals are clear statements of what you want out of life. They are most powerful when certain criteria are met (see fig. 3.1). It is important to word

FIGURE 3.1
Characteristics of Effective Goals

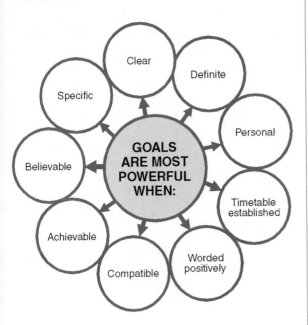

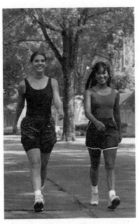

Associating with positive role models makes it easier for us to make health changes.

your goals in positive terms and have a specific timetable for their achievement. Goals motivate most effectively when they are your own personal goals that represent *your* desires, not goals that someone else has set for you.

It is important to have long-term goals that give direction to your life, and short-term goals that can serve as milestone achievements along the way. Here is an example of a long-term goal: By the end of six months, I will be able to walk at a comfortable but brisk pace for thirty minutes five times a week. An example of short-term goal is: For the next month, I will walk at a comfortable pace for thirty minutes three times a week.

Our current behavior and our success to change our behavior is influenced by family, friends, and others we associate with. People influence us by what they say, write, think, and by how they act. These influences can be both positive and negative. When the driver buckles a safety belt, the passengers often do the same. If we have friends who overeat, we have more of a tendency to stuff ourselves, too. We learn a great deal from others, and they learn from us. When we associate with people who exhibit healthy behaviors, it becomes easier for us to make positive changes. Of course, the opposite is also true.

STEPS TO CHANGE BEHAVIORS

Your success will be linked to developing and working on a systematic plan for change. This plan in-

TABLE 3.1
Steps to Change Behaviors

1.	**Identification**	Determine the most important behavior to change at this time.
2.	**Observation**	Become aware of the thoughts, feelings, and events that occur before and after the behavior you want to change.
3.	**Planning**	Determine a plan of action to replace your unhealthy behavior with a healthy one.
4.	**Monitoring**	Review your results and revise as necessary.

cludes four major steps that will help you reach your goal (see table 3.1).

Identification

What new behavior would you like for yourself? The behavior you choose depends entirely on you and on what you would like to improve about yourself. Most people already know the behaviors that are their strengths and those that are in need of change. Experts recommend changing only one behavior at a time. Giving your full attention and energy to one change increases your chance of success. The behavior you choose to focus on is called your **target behavior.**

To make it easier to make a change, adopt a new behavior to take the place of the unhealthy behavior. It is easier to think about adopting a new behavior rather than simply eliminating a less desirable one. The person who is ready to light a cigarette must place a target behavior, like reading a book, in its place. Otherwise, the sensed need to smoke that cigarette may be so strong that the person lights up.

Observation

"**Why should I observe and record my behavior, when I already know what I'm doing?**" is a question participants of behavior change programs often ask. Most of us think we understand why we behave the way we do. We also believe we can remember our past behavior. One study found that many people underreport how many calories they consume and overreport how much exercise they get. Also, many people cannot even remember the food they ate just two days ago. It is often easy to forget small, seemingly insignificant actions related to our behavior. But these patterns provide important clues. Observing and recording our actions provides factual information for our exact behaviors. It also provides insights into what we need to do to change. You can either record your actions yourself or ask someone to observe you; a combination of both often works best.

A journal is one of the best ways you can become aware of the situations, people, events, thoughts, and feelings that trigger your behavior. A journal is a record of the behaviors you engage in after some situation or event occurs. From it, you can keep track of the **antecedents** (the thoughts, actions, and events that occur before the behavior) and **consequences** (the events, feelings, and actions that occur after the behavior). Once you identify your antecedents and your consequences, you'll be better able to determine what needs to be changed. Changing your antecedents and your consequences also serves to change your behavior.

To record these antecedents and consequences, you'll need to make a note of the events that occur before and after the behavior. Suggestions to help identify antecedents and consequences are found in table 3.2. Each of these statements can be written on a small handheld notepad. It is best to take notes of the situation soon after it happens rather than to wait until the end of the day.

Careful self-observation will bring you many rewards and personal discoveries. Your journal will help you identify which situations influence your behavior. For example, a student wondered why she bit her nails. By using the behavioral diary, she found that she bit her nails when she was bored, angry, excited, stressed, or depressed; when watching TV, studying, or driving; and with certain people. The monitoring helped in understanding why she bit her nails and gave her a number of ideas for changing.

Thoughts and feelings should be monitored because they often precede and determine our actions. People often say they do not have control over how they feel about things. If they are not "tuned in" to their self-talk, they may not even be aware of their feelings. The truth is that we feel the way we do because of what we tell ourselves. How do we become aware of our

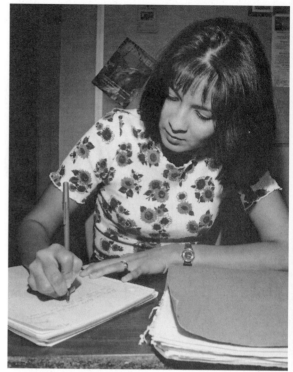

Keeping a journal will provide insights into what you need to make a change.

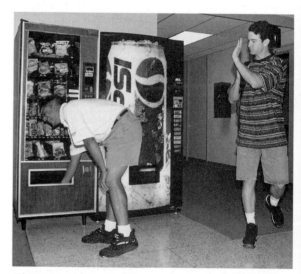

Change your antecedents to change your behavior.

self-talk? One way is to stand in front of a mirror and tell yourself that you are a wonderful human being, deserving of all the good things life has to offer. Listen to what you hear back from your "mirror self."

To understand how thoughts can lead to unhealthy behaviors, let's examine a sequence of thought patterns. You arrive home and have nothing to do. You tell yourself you feel bored and want to do something. Your attention turns to the kitchen and before

TABLE 3.2

Suggestions to Help Identify Antecedents and Consequences (Example is given for drinking and driving.)

Antecedents	Example
1. Where the behavior happened	On the way home from a party
2. When it happened	At midnight
3. Who were you with	Friends
4. What you were doing	Driving under the influence of alcohol (DUI)
5. What were you thinking	I'm drunk; hope I don't hit anybody
6. What you were feeling	Scared; I shouldn't be doing this

Consequences	Example
1. What happened afterward	Arrested for DUI
2. How you felt	Embarrassed; I deserved this
3. How you reacted	Passively
4. How others reacted	Laughed; ridiculed me
5. Outcome: positive, negative	Definitely negative and costly

you know it, your eyes are searching for something to eat (even though you are not hungry). You consume the snack and, within minutes, are bored once again. (Food has a limited capacity to relieve emotional discomfort such as boredom, because it is only effective for the time during which the person is eating.) You could choose to continue eating to relieve boredom or you could choose a healthy behavior, such as exercising, calling a friend, or studying. The series of thoughts in this example is termed a **behavior chain.** Fortunately, in most behavior chains, an individual can prevent a behavior chain from being cyclical at several intervention points (see fig. 3.2).

While thoughts are generally recorded using brief notes, feelings are often measured on a Likert scale. This is a scale on which you simply select your relative position, often between two extremes. For example, a student wanted to decrease his urges for a cigarette. To record his feelings, he made a Likert scale numbered from 1 to 10, where 1 represented no urge for a cigarette and 10 represented the most intense craving for one.

When people define success, many of them don't believe they have been successful at behavior changes unless they have completely reached their target goal. For example, a student who wanted to exercise five times a week for a month felt unsuccessful with her behavior change program because she was only able to jog an average of three times a week. Even though her target goal was not reached, numerous gains were still made. The key is that whether or not you have reached your target goal, you have achieved other benefits (see table 3.3).

FIGURE 3.2

Sample Behavior Chain

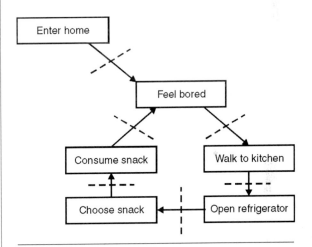

Each dotted line represents a decision point—an opportunity for alternative actions.

TABLE 3.3

Benefits Received from Attempting Behavior Change

1. Increased understanding of personal temptations
2. Increased feelings of self-control
3. Increased awareness of feeling and urges
4. Making friends with others trying the same project
5. Increased sensitivity toward others attempting health changes
6. Being able to forgive yourself when giving into temptation

FIGURE 3.3

Techniques for Changing Health Behaviors

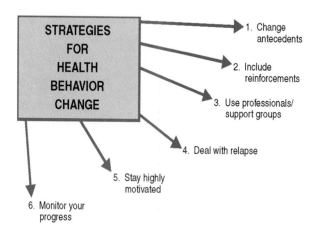

Although it is important to have high expectations, we need to realize that behavior change is a long-term process with challenges along the way. Sometimes changes come quickly, such as a smoker who successfully goes cold turkey. At other times changes come only after months of work, such as learning to vent anger constructively. When we document and measure these changes through our journal, we can feel much better about our own success—regardless of whether we have reached our predetermined goal.

Planning

After collecting information from your journal, you may find it easier to identify which techniques are needed to adopt your target behavior. A successful plan includes six strategies, which are highlighted in figure 3.3.

1. Change Antecedents

The thoughts, actions, and events (antecedents) that can occur before the unwanted behavior may help to trigger a new behavior. For example, one student kept her aerobic shoes in front of her door. This cue reminded her to exercise instead of watch TV when she came home. Another student, who had chosen to shed a few inches around the midsection, decided it was in his best interests to stop carrying change in his pockets. He couldn't resist eating the high-fat, high-calorie snacks from campus vending machines.

It is also important to change thought patterns that lead to unhealthy behaviors. Here is an example: A person who begins an exercise program is leaning toward skipping today's planned workout. He might have the thought, "It's okay to skip this day, I'll make sure to exercise tomorrow." To change this thought, he can tell himself, "Come on, let's go, you'll be glad you did."

2. Include Reinforcements

Rewards are very important in the early stages of behavior development. These rewards should be relatively easy to receive soon after the behavior is performed. You will be able to receive small rewards more often if you break down your large goal to smaller subgoals.

For some people, tangible rewards (e.g., money, clothing) are necessary. For others, the knowledge and enjoyment of completing a task are reward enough for the effort. Using both types of rewards can be especially powerful.

For some behaviors you can establish the type of reinforcements that Premack found to be effective. This involves using an enjoyable everyday activity as a reinforcer. Examples include eating dessert, driving, napping, watching TV, petting the dog or cat, and calling a friend. The rule is that you refrain from these enjoyable activities until you have performed your target behavior.

Self-reinforcement is another easy way to reward your efforts. Simply provide mental pats on the back after you accomplish a small goal along the way. Telling yourself "Good job, way to go" and "I knew you could do it!" are examples of self-reinforcement.

3. Use Professionals or a Support Group

We profit by allowing others to support us with our health behavior change. Professionals such as certified fitness instructors or dietitians can offer valuable assistance in overcoming unhealthy habits. You can also enlist your family, friends, teachers, and others who are willing to offer support. One idea is to have a friend join you who also wants to change the

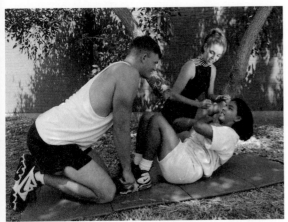

Support from others is another potent reinforcer for health behavior.

TABLE 3.4
High-Risk Situations for Relapse

1. Sickness
2. Accidents
3. "Weak moments"
4. Negative moods
5. Tempting social situations
6. Stress (anxiety)
7. Travel
8. Using alcohol and drugs
9. Fatigue
10. Relocating

same behavior. Bringing on a teammate allows both of you to encourage, motivate, and support each other. Or join a support group such as Overeaters Anonymous or Weight Watchers. Being with others who are working on the same behavior can provide that extra incentive for success.

We can also model ourselves after the health behavior of others, looking upon them as **role models.** Being around a friend or family member who is already practicing the desired behavior (i.e., exercise, healthy diet) can make it easier for us to make the change also.

4. Deal with Relapse

Relapse, or returning to an undesired behavior pattern, is a normal process for change. Even when we are totally committed to change and have a great start on our behavior change program, we may have a relapse and return to our old ways. Often, high-risk situations can lead to a relapse experience (see table 3.4).

A relapse is merely a temporary **setback to an old behavior pattern and does not mean you were unsuccessful with your behavior change effort.** If you happen to have a relapse, keep your mental spirits high. Realize that returning to old behaviors is a common experience that can provide you with useful information about yourself. For example, many smokers are not successful in quitting until they have relapsed five or more times. Each time a relapse occurs, they learn more about themselves and what it takes to be tobacco-free.

Relapses, for the most part, can be avoided if we plan and anticipate high-risk situations. Decide what actions you will take if you find yourself in a high-risk setting. Use visualization to imagine the tempting situation and observe yourself successfully working through the experience.

5. Stay Highly Motivated

If you find yourself returning to your old behavior patterns, be patient, stay focused, and keep in mind why you're making the change in the first place. Consider the following strategies to stay highly motivated:

- **Write a list of your reasons for making the behavior change.** Your reasons might include: to improve the quality and quantity of life, feel better, look better, have a better attitude, and so on. Post the list in a conspicuous place (mirror, wall, bulletin board, or refrigerator) where you can see it daily.
- **Complete a behavioral contract.** Your contract should include when you will begin your project and provide subgoals you expect to reach as you move toward your final target behavior. It is often witnessed by a friend or colleague. A sample contract is provided in Activity 3 at the end of this chapter.
- **Visualize yourself after you have reached your goal.** The mind is a powerful tool to change your behavior. Through visualization, you can program your mind (like programming a computer) to carry out your mission. Close your eyes and see yourself the "way you want to be" after reaching your target behavior. For example, if your goal is to lose weight and fat, admire your new figure. In your mind's eye, notice how well the clothes fit on your body. Cherish the smile on your slimmer face.

6. Monitor Your Progress

The last strategy to change behavior is to monitor your progress. The next section provides a detailed description of monitoring and its importance to the success of a behavior change.

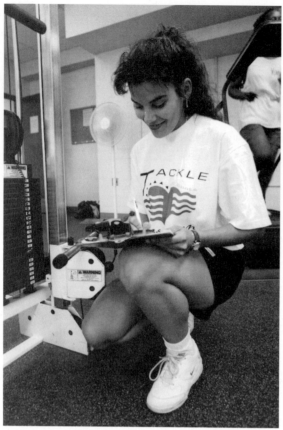

Documenting your performance will allow you to stay on task and reach your goals.

Monitoring

To change a behavior successfully, it is important to have a monitoring system. Keeping a journal, log, graph, chart, or tape recording of your voice are the common methods for monitoring behavior. Documenting your performance will allow you to stay on task and reach your target behavior. When you record your results on paper, you receive feedback about your performance. One student charted how many miles she walked in one month. She was surprised to discover that she had walked sixty total miles.

Through your monitoring system, you may find that your initial plan is not working as you first imagined. If your subgoals are too easy or too difficult to attain, you can become easily discouraged. In either case, change your subgoals so that they will work for you. And, as you begin reaching them, make sure to reward yourself. This will encourage you to keep on track.

Regardless of whether or not you reach your target behavior, keep in mind that you are still a winner. If we could easily change ourselves, everyone would have a high level of success. Unfortunately, to make changes in our behavior can be and often is a challenging and frustrating experience. In fact, many people avoid making changes altogether, even when ordered to by their physician. And of those who do try, many become discouraged and falter.

It is hoped this chapter has equipped you with the knowledge and skills necessary to make health and fitness changes. When you reverse your unhealthy patterns, you can take pride in knowing you are moving toward a higher level of well-being.

SUMMARY

- Behaviors are the physical and psychological actions that are performed in response to some type of stimuli.
- In most cases, our goals, personal values, beliefs, knowledge, attitudes, and unmet needs drive us. And often we are motivated by other individuals—we want to behave in ways we feel are expected of us.
- Goals are clear statements of what we want out of life and are important to making health changes.
- The four major steps for changing health behaviors are identification, observation, planning, and monitoring.
- A journal is one of the best ways to become aware of the situations, people, events, thoughts, and feelings that influence health behavior.
- Success in attempting health changes can be measured in other gains besides reaching the target behavior. Two include increased understanding of personal temptations and increased awareness of feelings and urges.
- The six strategies for changing health behaviors are (1) change the antecedents, (2) include reinforcements, (3) use professionals or a support group, (4) deal with relapse, (5) stay highly motivated, and (6) monitor progress.
- Your personal commitment to change will bring the reward of an increased sense of personal control, plus the buoyant feeling of being healthier. You have the power to change your behavioral patterns—the ball is in your court.

ACTIVITY 3

HEALTH BEHAVIOR CHANGE CONTRACT

Name _____   **To be submitted: Yes   No**

Date _____   **If yes, due date** _____

Class _____   **Section** _____   **Score** _____

PURPOSE
1. To use a behavioral contract in making a health change.
2. To get off to a great start so that the new behavior is adopted as part of your daily routine.
3. To get a "feel" of an instrument you can use with your support-team participants to change your health behavior.

DIRECTIONS
1. Decide on a behavior you are committed to change. Whether you decide to adopt (e.g., fitness program), modify (e.g., lose weight), or eliminate (e.g., smoking) a health behavior, making out a contract will help ensure your success. An exercise program is used as an example.
2. Answer the questions on the health change contract.
3. Stay with the contract a minimum of 3 weeks. For most people, it takes at least 21 days for a new behavior to become a normal part of their lifestyle.
4. After the minimum 3-week period, answer the questions in the Results section of this lab.

HEALTH CHANGE CONTRACT
(3 points each except for #12, which is worth 15 points)

1. Specific behavior I want to change: (e.g., become physically fit)

   _____

2. It is important for me to be successful with this change because I want to: (e.g., live longer, look and feel better, and reduce my risk of disease).

   a. _____

   b. _____

   c. _____

3. Specific outcomes expected as a result of making the change: (e.g., lose 4 pounds, reduce waistline by 2 inches, exercise for 30 minutes without stopping).

   a. _____

   b. _____

   c. _____

4. My subgoals for each week are: (e.g., 1st week: walk 1 mile, 2nd week: walk 1 1/4 miles, 3rd week: walk 1 1/2 miles).

   Week 1: _____

   Week 2: _____

   Week 3: _____

5. My plan of action to carry out this health change will be to: (e.g., include stretching, weights, and a walking program 5 days a week).

   _____

   _____

6. I plan to use a daily (diary, log, graph, or chart) to monitor my successful performance. _____

7. Barriers I will face and strategies to overcome them. For example, if time is a barrier, your strategies could be to exercise at lunch or wake up earlier.

    Barriers   *Strategies*

    a. _____   a. _____

    b. _____   b. _____

    c. _____   c. _____

8. The following people have agreed to be on my support team:

    a. _____

    b. _____

    c. _____

9. When I am successful, I will reward myself by: (e.g., a pat on the back, new clothes, new shoes).

    a. _____

    b. _____

    c. _____

10. I plan to start this behavior change on _____ (date) and will stay with it for _____ weeks.

11. I estimate my chances of success to be (0–100%) _____.

12. In a paragraph, cite a minimum of three references related to your health behavior change. Use information from these references to assist you in "why" to make the health change and the "how" to actually make the change. Include a bibliography in this section.

13. You signature _____

    Witness _____

RESULTS

1. Were you successful in your attempted behavior change?
   Yes   No   Explain.

2. If you were to attempt this change again, what would you do differently, if anything? Explain.

3. If you were to tackle another health change, what would it be? When would you begin?

4. What were your honest thoughts about going through this process of changing health behaviors? Was this a valuable experience for you? Yes, No, Why, or Why Not?

2

STRATEGIES FOR A SAFE AND EFFECTIVE FITNESS PROGRAM

4

STRATEGIES TO PLAN FOR FITNESS

To receive optimal benefits, use proper strategies to exercise effectively!

LEARNING OBJECTIVES

- Determine whether you need medical clearance before starting an exercise program.

- Describe the proper strategies to exercise effectively.

- Examine the importance of the warm-up and cooldown.

- Identify the proper clothing and footwear for a year-round physical fitness program.

- Design a personal physical fitness program.

LIFESTYLE QUESTIONS

- Are you in good enough health to participate in a physical fitness program?

- Have you ever properly designed a physical fitness program for yourself?

- Do you own the proper clothing and footwear to exercise year-round?

- Do you believe planning would motivate you to start and maintain your own fitness program?

INTRODUCTION

Beginning your own fitness program can be exciting and challenging. As you already know, being fit has many benefits. As with most things in life, there are correct ways and incorrect ways to go about becoming fit. This chapter provides you with strategies for the best way to have a successful fitness program. Smart planning is the key to your enjoyment, safety, and success in your lifetime personal fitness program.

MEDICAL READINESS

To be on the safe side, it is important to be medically cleared before starting any fitness program. Although exercise generally is considered a safe activity, it is wise to assess your medical history by identifying any preexisting medical conditions before starting a fitness program. In addition to identifying any present health problems, doctors believe the key to a physical is taking a family history and assessing your lifestyle. The fact that you have gained weight

and rarely exercise may be particularly relevant if you also report a family history of diabetes and high blood pressure. Likewise, if you're a young adult and your grandparents died of heart disease, your doctor might order tests now to check your cholesterol and lipid levels instead of waiting for you to get much older.

Chances are you'll be given a clean bill of health, but it still is in your best interests to receive the official clearance. Although a physical is not 100 percent foolproof, getting the green light from your physician is the sure way to verify your readiness for exercise. Fill out the questionnaire in Activity 4A to determine whether you are medically ready to participate in a physical fitness program.

EFFECTIVE EXERCISE STRATEGIES

Careful attention to effective exercise strategies will help ensure safety and maximize results from your fitness program (see fig. 4.1).

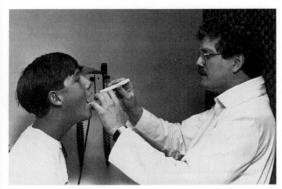

A physical examination is important before starting an exercise program.

FIGURE 4.1
Effective Exercise Strategies

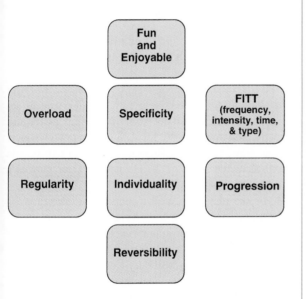

Fun and Enjoyable

If you enjoy a particular activity like swimming and have fun doing it, you are more likely to engage in it. Like anything else, what you enjoy doing, you'll do, and what you don't enjoy, you'll try and get out of. Over the long run, enjoying your exercise is one of the most important strategies for a successful program. What's important to a year-round, lifetime fitness program is that you choose activities that are fun and that you look forward to participating in. If you ever get to the point where exercise becomes "work" and you don't look forward to it, then it's time to switch to new activities that are stimulating and enjoyable.

Overload

For a muscle or system to become stronger, it must be overloaded or taken beyond its normal limits. To strengthen your heart muscle, for example, you must gradually work it beyond its normal workload. If you exercise at a brisk pace, you will stimulate your heart to work harder than normal. This, in turn, will promote a stronger and healthier heart muscle. The same is true for all muscles and systems of the body.

Once a muscle adapts to a higher workload, further gains in fitness require additional increases in workload. To maintain an adequate level of fitness, a normal amount of exercise is recommended. If the overload is below normal for a health-related component, there will be a decline of fitness in that specific component. Also, even though gradual overloading is essential for becoming fit, you don't want to place too much overload or stress at any one time. This can lead to pain and damage or injury to the body.

Specificity

To develop a certain level of fitness in a health-related component, you must overload specifically for that fitness component. For example, if you want to improve cardiorespiratory fitness, you must choose activities such as brisk walking, jogging, bicycling, swimming, and dancing that are specific to heart and lung function.

Progression

The three methods to progress from your current level of fitness are to gradually increase: (1) frequency, (2) intensity, and/or (3) time of exercise. Whichever method or methods you choose, remember to stay within recommended guidelines. If you exercise too often, too hard, and too long, it can be hazardous to your health and lead to burnout, frustration, and quitting your program—exactly what you don't want to happen! Participating infrequently in high-intensity exercise can be dangerous. The basketball player who plays competitively only on the weekends is a good example. Exercising as a weekend warrior can lead to muscle soreness, injury, and heat-related disorders.

Frequency, Intensity, Time, and Type (FITT)

A brief description of the FITT formula is addressed in this section. A more thorough discussion of each guideline and how it applies to the five components of health-related fitness can be found in chapters 5 to 8.

Frequency (How Often)

For exercise to be most effective, it must be performed on a regular basis year-round. Experts recommend three to seven days a week (depending on the intensity of the activity) for improving the components of health-related fitness.

FIGURE 4.2

Exercise in your fitness target zone to receive maximum benefits.

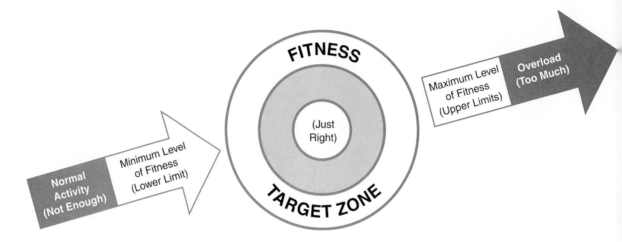

Intensity (How Hard)

For exercise to be most effective, it must be performed vigorously enough to require the body to exert more effort than usual. The additional workload will lead to improvement in health-related fitness.

Exercise becomes most effective when the fitness target zone is reached for all five health-related components (see fig. 4.2). Each health-related component has its own fitness target zone. Running faster than normal for cardiorespiratory fitness and stretching beyond normal limits for flexibility are examples of increasing the workload to produce fitness gains.

Time (How Long)

Experts recommend twenty to sixty minutes of continuous exercise to receive health and fitness benefits. If you are beginning a fitness program, start with shorter time sessions and gradually add time to your workouts as your fitness level improves. Most health and fitness benefits can be derived by accumulating at least thirty minutes or more of physical activity (time spent can be continuous or in bouts of at least ten minutes provided it totals thirty minutes per day).

Type (What Kind)

Experts agree that aerobic exercise is particularly effective for cardiorespiratory endurance and reducing body fat. Aerobic exercises are activities in which the body is able to supply sufficient oxygen to the working muscles for long periods of time. Choosing aerobic exercises you enjoy is important for maintaining a regular program. Walking, jogging, swimming, dancing, bicycling, and cross-country skiing are excellent forms of aerobic exercise. However, these exercises do not promote total fitness because they do not target each of the five health-related components.

Adding flexibility and strength-training exercises would provide a well-rounded fitness program.

Individuality

In planning your exercise program, make sure to select activities that meet your individual goals and needs. See Activity 4C for designing your own personal fitness program. Remember that no two people will have the same goals and needs. Your partner's fitness program may be entirely different from yours. He or she may only want to pursue cardiorespiratory endurance while you may have as your goal to increase both cardiorespiratory endurance and muscular strength. Plus, individuals respond differently to exercise, and adaptations will vary from one person to another. For example, you may take less time to develop cardiorespiratory fitness than your partner does.

Regularity

A major roadblock with starting a fitness program is finding time in an already busy schedule. Chances are you already have many demands placed on your time, including classes, homework, test and term paper preparation, work schedules, family responsibilities, and so on. Nonetheless, it is important to schedule a time for activity on most, if not all, days and stick to it.

Some people like to exercise first thing in the morning—it helps them get ready for the day; some people like to exercise at lunch time—it helps them break up their day; and still others like to work out in the evening—it helps them remove the stress that has accumulated throughout the day. The best time for you is when you are most motivated to do it and that time is available. The key in starting is to be consistent with exercise until it is part of your daily routine. After exercise becomes a regular part of your life, chances are you won't be able to live without it!

Reversibility

The benefits of being physically fit will only stay with you as long as you exercise. If you ever stop, the benefits you enjoyed will stop too. Generally, physiological changes begin to reverse if a person is inactive for a period of forty-eight hours or longer. With inactivity, muscles weaken, joints lose their range of motion, the resting heart rate rises, and the composition of your body begins to shift toward a greater percentage of fat tissue. It is important to stay active and remain fit to continue enjoying the health benefits and avoid the changes associated with reversibility.

WARM-UP AND COOLDOWN

The three important parts of an exercise session are the warm-up, actual workout, and cooldown. Besides the workout, the warm-up and the cooldown are highly recommended each time you exercise. Although many exercisers spend little or no time warming up and cooling down, experts agree they are important parts of your total workout.

Warm-Up

A good warm-up offers numerous benefits to the exerciser. It prepares the muscles and heart for the exercise workout. Warming up can also improve your performance and reduce your risk of injury. It does this by increasing muscle temperature and allowing your heart rate to increase gradually. Vigorous stretching of cold muscles can result in muscle soreness and injury. A slow elevation in heart rate is a safety measure to avoid unnecessary cardiac strain.

The warm-up period is also a time to prepare your mind for exercise. The warm-up is a time to think about your fitness goals and what you need to do during this exercise session to achieve those goals. Exercise can be more enjoyable and effective if you have the proper mental attitude for your workout.

There are different approaches to the warm-up. The traditional method of warming up is to perform gentle, static stretching first (see chapter 7). This is followed by a slower form of your chosen exercise, whether it be walking, jogging, dancing, and so on. The other method now recommended is to move your body slowly for two to five minutes to warm the muscles and joints before stretching. The key to warming up is to start slowly, and gradually warm up before vigorous activity.

The proper warm-up will require at least five to ten minutes and prepare you physically and mentally for the more vigorous portion of your workout.

Cooldown

The cooldown is often the most neglected portion of a workout. From a safety standpoint, the cooldown is essential to your regular fitness program. The purpose of the cooldown is to let the body return to its normal functioning level. If performed correctly, the cooldown maintains a moderate heart rate and venous blood flow, which facilitates the removal of waste products from muscle tissue. This allows a faster and more complete recovery.

A danger of an improper cooldown is blood pooling. During exercise, the heart pumps blood and needed oxygen to the working muscles. This action keeps the muscles moving. As the muscles contract rhythmically during exercise, the veins are alternately squeezed and released. This milking action forces the blood in your veins to move toward your heart. One-way valves and blood pressure prevent the blood from flowing in the other direction.

If you stop exercising abruptly and do not cooldown properly, the muscle contractions in the legs also stop. Blood tends to pool in your veins, especially in your legs. A lack of venous blood return from the legs can result in a lack of oxygen to the brain. This can cause dizziness and blackout.

Like the warm-up, the cooldown should consist of a slower activity and gentle, static stretching. The best way to cooldown and prevent health problems is to slowly taper off or gradually reduce your speed immediately after the aerobic workout. Next, gentle, static stretching is recommended.

The amount of time spent cooling down will depend on how vigorously you worked out and your level of fitness. Generally, the cooldown should last five to ten minutes. Of this, at least two minutes should be devoted to reducing your speed and slowing down. Stretching exercises can make up the rest of the time. The same stretching exercises for the warm-up can also be used for the cooldown.

A SAMPLE WARM-UP AND COOLDOWN PROGRAM

(Stretch to a point of mild discomfort and hold all stretches for at least ten seconds.)

1. **The Posterior Shoulder Stretch.** Start in a standing position. Place your right arm overhead with your elbow bent. Grasp your right elbow with your left hand and gently pull your right elbow and upper arm behind your head. Hold this position. Repeat this exercise with the left arm.
2. **Side Stretch.** Stand with your feet shoulder-width apart. Place both arms straight above your head, grabbing one hand with the other. Lean to

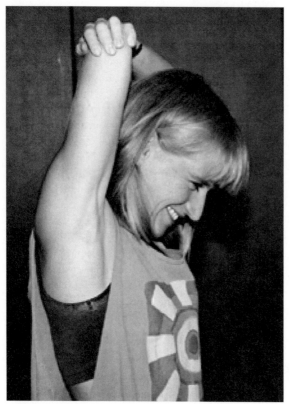

Posterior shoulder stretch

the left. Stretch all of the muscles along the right side of your body. Hold this position. Repeat this exercise leaning to the right.

3. **Low Back Stretch.** Start in a position lying on your back with both legs straight. Pull one thigh toward your chest with your knee bent and both hands behind your thigh. Hold this position. Repeat this exercise using the opposite leg.

4. **Lunge Stretch.** From a standing position take a large step forward. Bend the knee of your forward leg. Keep your feet pointed straight ahead. With your upper body erect and your arms out to the sides for balance, slowly press down and forward with your hips, stretching the muscles that cross the front of the hip joint. Bring your arms back, stretching the shoulder muscles at the same time. Hold this position. Repeat this exercise using the opposite leg.

5. **Calf Stretch.** Stand facing a wall approximately three feet away with your feet about twelve inches apart. Lean forward from the ankles and place your hands on the wall. Keep your body and your legs straight. Lean forward as far as possible while keeping your feet flat on the floor. Hold this position.

6. **The Cardiorespiratory Warm-Up and Cooldown.** Before and after vigorous exercise, slowly perform your aerobic workout for a minimum of

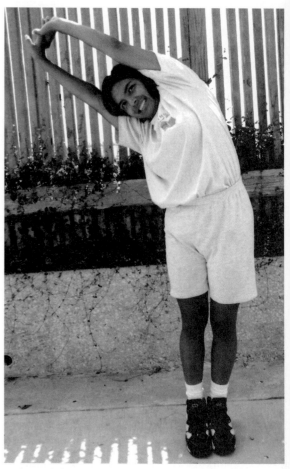

Side stretch

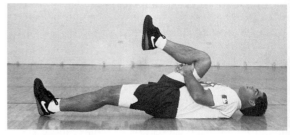

Low back stretch

two minutes. Two common warm-up and cooldown activities are walking and slow jogging.

CLOTHING AND PROPER FOOTWEAR

The proper exercise clothing is important for year-round participation. Although fashion looks good, comfort should be given top priority for exercise clothing. Your clothes should be comfortable and not confining. As the seasons change, so do the clothes. The clothing you wear should also be appropriate for

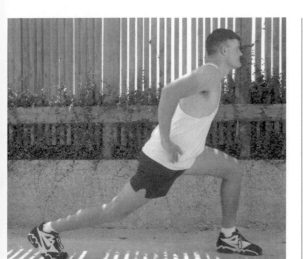

Lunge stretch

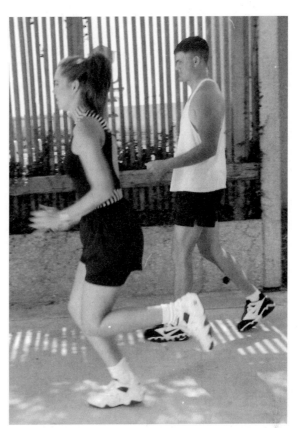

Two common warm-up and cooldown activities are slow jogging and walking.

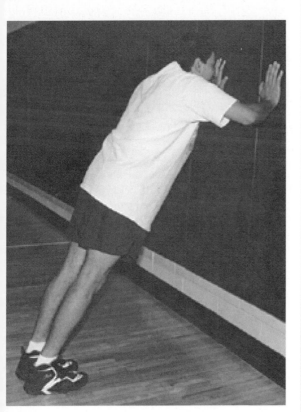

Calf stretch

your exercise. Ideally, the clothing closest to the skin should be breathable, allowing for sweat evaporation. Exercise bras and athletic supporters will provide firm support and make exercise more comfortable.

For hot weather, wear light-colored, light-weight, and loose-fitting clothing. Light-colored clothing reflects some of the sun's rays and light-weight clothing will not add unnecessary weight to your body. Loose-fitting clothing will allow air to cir-

culate next to your skin. All three of these will keep you cooler on a hot day. For sunny weather, a hat and sunglasses will help prevent headaches and fatigue.

For exercising in cold weather, wear layers of clothing with a woolen hat and mittens. Layers of clothing will allow you to regulate body temperature as you exercise. A warm-up suit over other exercise clothing is preferred because it can be removed if desired. In cold weather, it is also important to cover your head with a woolen hat and your hands with gloves or mittens. As much as 70 percent of your body heat can be lost from your head and hands if they are not covered.

Appropriate footwear is vital for most fitness activities. Shoe companies now have a shoe for just about every activity. Whether it is walking, jogging, bicycling, dance, or water aerobics, there is a shoe made specifically for that activity. For safety and performance, purchase shoes designed specifically for your planned activity.

When shopping for exercise shoes, be a good comparison shopper. It is wise to spend a little extra time and money to get a shoe with good quality and a comfortable fit. A final note—many exercisers wait too long before replacing worn-out shoes. Purchase a new pair of shoes either when the midsole has lost its resiliency or when the outer sole has worn out.

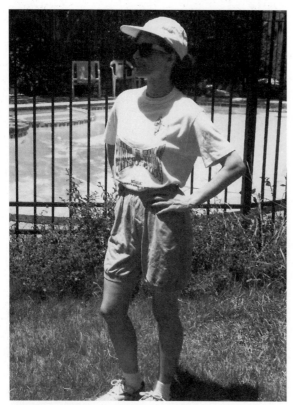

Wear light-colored, loose-fitting, and lightweight clothing when exercising in hot weather.

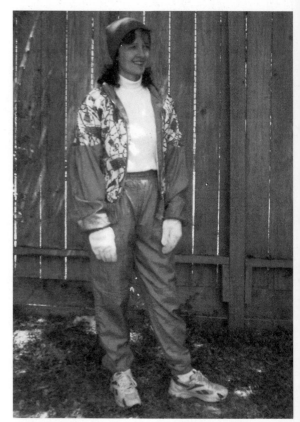

Dress in layers for exercising in cold weather.

SUMMARY

- Smart planning is the key to your enjoyment, safety, and success in your lifetime personal fitness program.
- To be on the safe side, it is important to be medically cleared before starting any fitness program.
- Careful attention to effective exercise strategies will help ensure safety and maximize results from your fitness program.
- The eight strategies are: (1) fun and enjoyable, (2) overload, (3) specificity, (4) progression, (5) frequency, intensity, time, and type (FITT), (6) individuality, (7) regularity, and (8) reversibility.
- A good warm-up offers numerous benefits to the exerciser. It prepares the muscles and heart for the exercise workout, improves performance, reduces risk of injury, and prepares the mind for exercise.
- There are different approaches to the warm-up. The traditional method is to perform gentle, static stretching first. This is followed by a slower form of your chosen exercise. The other method is to first move your body slowly for two to five minutes before stretching. The key is to start slowly and gradually warm up before vigorous activity.
- From a safety standpoint, the cooldown is essential to your regular fitness program. The purpose

of the cooldown is to let the body return to its normal functioning level. If performed correctly, the cooldown maintains a moderate heart rate and venous blood flow, which facilitates the removal of waste products from muscle tissue. This allows a faster and more complete recovery.
- Like the warm-up, the cooldown should consist of a slower activity and gentle, static stretching. The best way to cooldown and prevent health problems is to slowly taper off or gradually reduce your speed immediately after the aerobic workout. Next, gentle, static stretching is recommended.
- The proper exercise clothing is important for year-round participation. Although fashion looks good, comfort should be given top priority for exercise clothing.
- For hot weather, wear light-colored, lightweight, and loose-fitting clothing.
- For exercising in cold weather, wear layers of clothing with a woolen hat and mittens. Layers of clothing will allow you to regulate body temperature as you exercise.
- Appropriate footwear is vital for most fitness activities. When shopping for exercise shoes, be a good comparison shopper. Also, replace exercise shoes often to prevent injury.

A C T I V I T Y   4A
THE MEDICAL CLEARANCE QUESTIONNAIRE

Name _____   To be submitted: Yes   No

Date _____   If yes, due date _____

Class _____   Section _____   Score _____

PURPOSE
To determine if you are medically ready to participate in an exercise program.

DIRECTIONS
1. Circle either yes or no for each of the questions in the questionnaire.
2. Answer the questions in the Results section.

MEDICAL CLEARANCE QUESTIONNAIRE
1. Yes   No   Are you over 35 years of age?
2. Yes   No   Do you have any type of heart or blood vessel disease?
3. Yes   No   Do you have high blood pressure?
4. Yes   No   Do you ever experience chest pain?
5. Yes   No   Do you ever experience breathlessness?
6. Yes   No   Do you have any bone or joint problems?
7. Yes   No   Do you ever feel faint or dizzy?
8. Yes   No   Are you a smoker?
9. Yes   No   Have you been inactive for the last two years?
10. Yes   No   Do you have a weight problem?
11. Yes   No   Do you have any medical condition that could be a problem if you started exercising?

Note: If you responded with a yes to any of the questions, or if you have any doubt about your health, get medical clearance from your physician before starting an exercise program. It is also a good idea to let your instructor know what questions you answered yes to.

RESULTS
1. Did you answer yes to any of the questions in the medical questionnaire?   Yes   No   If so, which one(s)?

2. If you answered yes to any of the questions, does your physician know about your health status?

3. Do you feel healthy enough to begin or maintain an exercise program?

A C T I V I T Y   **4B**

THE WARM-UP AND COOLDOWN

Name _____   **To be submitted: Yes   No**

Date _____   **If yes, due date** _____

Class _____   **Section** _____   **Score** _____

PURPOSE
To acquaint you with suitable exercises for warming up and cooling down.

DIRECTIONS
Perform the exercises described in chapter 4 on pages 43 to 44.

RESULTS
1. Did you enjoy performing the different stretching exercises?   Yes   No

2. Do you feel the stretching exercises can serve as an effective warm-up and cooldown for your aerobic workout?   Yes   No

3. What are your future plans for warming up and cooling down? Check one.

    a. _____ I plan to warm up and cool down mainly when I exercise.

    b. _____ I plan to stretch daily, whether I exercise or not.

    c. _____ I plan to stretch like I have in the past—only when I get out of bed!

ACTIVITY   *4C*

DESIGNING YOUR PHYSICAL FITNESS PROGRAM

Name _____   **To be submitted: Yes   No**

Date _____   **If yes, due date** _____

Class _____ **Section** _____   **Score** _____

PURPOSE
To plan your own exercise program. A regular, effective, and year-round fitness program takes careful planning.

DIRECTIONS
Answer all questions in the following sections.

A. List several benefits you want to achieve from your personal fitness program (weight loss, more strength, less stress, etc.).

B. Circle your level of fitness related to the five components of health-related fitness.

Although you may not precisely know your levels of fitness, you probably have a good idea where you stand. For example, if you have been inactive, it's likely you have low levels of fitness in four (maybe not body composition) and maybe in all five health-related components.

HEALTH-RELATED COMPONENT	LEVEL OF FITNESS		
1. Cardiorespiratory Fitness	Low	Medium	High
2. Strength (Lower Body)	Low	Medium	High
(Upper Body)	Low	Medium	High
3. Muscular Endurance (Lower Body)	Low	Medium	High
(Upper Body)	Low	Medium	High
4. Flexibility	Low	Medium	High
5. Body Composition	Low	Medium	High

(Overfat usually indicates a low level of fitness.)

Name: _____

C. Looking back at your levels of fitness, choose activities that will best meet your fitness goals.

1. Cardiorespiratory Fitness

Activities _____ _____ _____

   (Walking, jogging, swimming, dancing, bicycling, basketball, racquetball, tennis, etc.)

   Goals   Length of workout _____ minutes

                  Workouts per week _____

2. Strength

Activities _____ _____ _____

   (Weight machines, free weights, push-ups, sit-ups, pull-ups, etc.)

   Goals   Length of workout _____ minutes

                  Workouts per week _____

3. Muscular Endurance

Activities _____ _____ _____

   (Same activities used for cardiorespiratory fitness and strength can be used for muscular endurance)

   Goals   Length of workout _____ minutes

                  Workouts per week _____

4. Flexibility

Activities _____ _____ _____

   (Static stretching, ballistic stretching, PNF) (see chapter 7)

   Goals   Length of workout _____ minutes

                  Workouts per week _____

5. Body Composition

Activities _____ _____ _____

   (Same activities used for cardiorespiratory fitness supplemented by strength and muscular endurance activities will work for body composition)

   Goals   Length of workout _____ minutes

                  Workouts per week _____

Name: _____

D. Plan a weekly exercise schedule by identifying the activities and times you plan to exercise this week.

Monday Activities	Times	Tuesday Activities	Times	Wednesday Activities	Times
Thursday Activities	Times	Friday Activities	Times	Saturday Activities	Times
Sunday Activities	Times				

RESULTS

1. Were you able to follow your weekly exercise schedule?   Yes   No

2. If yes, what are your thoughts about your exercise program?

3. If you did not participate in an exercise program, do you plan to begin one soon?   Yes   No

4. What are your future exercise plans?

STRATEGIES FOR CARDIORESPIRATORY ENDURANCE

Give your heart special care with exercise—it's the one muscle that better work well!

LEARNING OBJECTIVES

- Identify the characteristics necessary for cardiorespiratory endurance.

- Describe some of the major benefits of a cardiorespiratory fitness program.

- Explain the effective exercise strategies to develop cardiorespiratory endurance.

- Learn how to measure your heart rate and compute your estimated target heart rate range.

- Describe the two types of exercises and training methods used to develop and maintain cardiorespiratory endurance.

- Perform two fitness tests to measure cardiorespiratory endurance.

LIFESTYLE QUESTIONS

- Do you consider yourself to have a fit circulatory system that includes your heart muscle?

- Do you consider yourself to have a fit respiratory system?

- What is your resting heart rate?

- Would you like to improve your level of cardiorespiratory endurance?

INTRODUCTION

Physical fitness experts usually consider cardiorespiratory endurance to be the most important component of health-related fitness. Cardiorespiratory endurance has achieved its high status in the medical world because of its value in combating heart disease, strokes, high blood pressure, obesity, and stress. This component of fitness is also important to many types of work, play, and sports activities.

Cardiorespiratory endurance involves the capacity to continue vigorous total body activity for a relatively long period of time. It is the ability of your heart, lungs, blood vessels, and blood to effectively supply oxygen and nutrients to the working muscles while removing waste products. The heart and lungs are your primary organs associated with intake, delivery, and utilization of oxygen.

If you possess cardiorespiratory fitness, you can continue in vigorous activities such as brisk walking, jogging, swimming, bicycling, and dancing for pro-

longed periods of time. This is because you have efficient circulatory and respiratory systems. In some unconditioned individuals, the ability of the cardiorespiratory system may be so limited that climbing a flight of stairs or walking to class can cause shortness of breath and a rapid heartbeat.

CHARACTERISTICS FOR CARDIORESPIRATORY ENDURANCE

The following characteristics are necessary to achieve cardiorespiratory endurance.

Fit Heart Muscle
Like any other muscle, your heart must be regularly exercised to become stronger. When properly exercised, your heart becomes larger, stronger, and more efficient. The reverse is also true. A fit heart muscle can pump a greater amount of blood with less

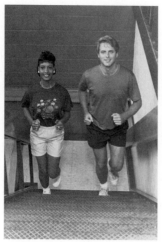

Climbing a flight of stairs is easier if you are physically fit.

beats per minute. For example, as a regular exerciser, you may have a resting heart rate in the low sixties, whereas an inactive person typically has a heart rate in the seventies or eighties.

Fit Blood Vessel System

Your heart and blood vessel system work in a very efficient manner. After servicing your body tissues, your blood returns to the right side of your heart, which pumps the blood to your lungs. There it is saturated with oxygen, returned to the left side of your heart, and then pumped to all parts of your body by the arterial systems (see fig. 5.1).

Your arteries divide into smaller and smaller branches, and finally into capillaries, the smallest blood vessels of all. The blood within the capillaries supplies oxygen and nutrients to your cells, and takes up your waste products. Your blood returns to your heart by your veins. Carbon dioxide and other waste materials are removed from your body by your lungs and kidneys.

The blood in the heart's four chambers does not directly nourish your heart. Rather, it is the many small coronary arteries within your heart muscle that supply the blood circulation to the heart. Insufficient blood circulation, hastened by unhealthy arteries, can lead to heart disease.

Regular physical exercise contributes to a healthy blood vessel system. It is especially important to maintain the health of your coronary arteries of the heart and the carotid arteries that lead to your brain. Both are susceptible to internal narrowing or fatty buildup (**atherosclerosis**) and a loss of elasticity or hardening (**arteriosclerosis**). These conditions can lead to heart attacks and strokes.

FIGURE 5.1

(a) Blood is supplied to heart tissues by branches of the coronary arteries. (b) Blood is drained from heart tissues by branches of the cardiac veins.

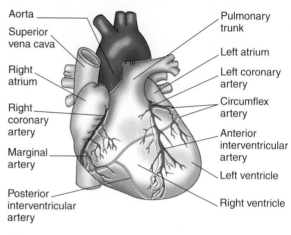

Aorta
Superior vena cava
Right atrium
Right coronary artery
Marginal artery
Posterior interventricular artery

Pulmonary trunk
Left atrium
Left coronary artery
Circumflex artery
Anterior interventricular artery
Left ventricle
Right ventricle

(a)

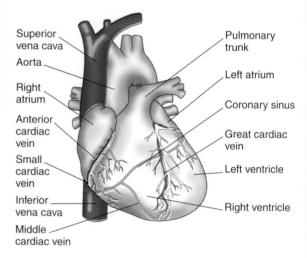

Superior vena cava
Aorta
Right atrium
Anterior cardiac vein
Small cardiac vein
Inferior vena cava
Middle cardiac vein

Pulmonary trunk
Left atrium
Coronary sinus
Great cardiac vein
Left ventricle
Right ventricle

(b)

Fit Respiratory System

Respiration is the process of exchanging gases between the atmosphere and your body's cells. External respiration is the process of inhaling oxygen and having it delivered to the lungs, where it is absorbed by the blood. This process requires fit lungs and red blood cells with sufficient levels of **hemoglobin** (the protein that carries iron and oxygen in the blood). **Anemia** is the condition in which there is insufficient supply of red blood cells with hemoglobin.

Internal respiration is delivering oxygen to your tissues from your blood. Both respiration processes also remove carbon dioxide, a waste product. If your blood vessels are not narrowed and there is a sufficient number of healthy capillaries, the exchange of gases will reach each individual cell.

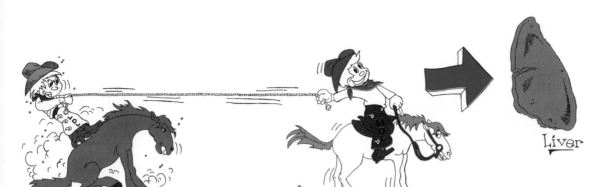

HDL (good cholesterol) acts as a scavenger to carry LDL (bad cholesterol) to the liver where it is metabolized.

Fit Blood

Having healthy blood is important for your fit cardiorespiratory system. Your blood transports nutrients, oxygen, hormones, and waste products. It also helps regulate your internal body temperature by picking up heat from deep body tissues and either distributing it throughout your body or taking it to your skin for elimination.

Your blood can carry oxygen effectively because its four to six billion red blood cells contain hemoglobin. Hemoglobin is composed of a protein (globin) and an iron-containing pigment (hematin) that can bind with oxygen.

Fit Muscle Tissue

Once the oxygen is delivered to your muscles, they must be able to use oxygen to maintain physical activity. If your muscle cells can utilize the oxygen effectively, you can continue your workout without fatigue or having to stop.

SOME MAJOR BENEFITS OF A CARDIORESPIRATORY FITNESS PROGRAM

When you participate in a cardiorespiratory fitness program with appropriate and sufficient frequency, intensity, and time (duration), your body can respond with the following positive changes:

1. A larger, stronger, and more efficient heart muscle (especially in the left ventricle).
2. An increase in stroke volume (the amount of blood pumped per beat).
3. A decrease in resting heart rate.
4. Healthier blood vessels. The blood-carrying capacity of the arteries improves because their muscular walls get stronger and increase in elasticity.
5. The lowering of mildly elevated blood pressure.

6. An increase in the number of capillaries that surround and service each muscle fiber. This enables more oxygen to diffuse to each muscle fiber, allowing you as an exerciser to work longer and recover faster than an untrained person.
7. Greater blood volume. This decreases thickness and the chance of blood clots that can cause heart attacks and strokes.
8. A reduction in low-density lipoproteins (LDL) and an increase in high-density lipoproteins (HDL). LDL is the type of fat (lipid) that attaches to the inside walls of the arteries and results in the narrowing of the arteries. HDL functions in a positive manner by collecting LDL from the bloodstream and carrying it to the liver for alterations and metabolism.
9. Improved breathing. Air can be moved in and out of the lungs with less effort.
10. Using up more calories. More than any other type of exercise, aerobic activities reduce weight and body fat.
11. An increase in bone strength and density.
12. An increase in mental benefits. Aerobic exercises can reduce stress, improve relaxation, and develop a more positive outlook toward life and self.

STRATEGIES FOR CARDIORESPIRATORY ENDURANCE

To develop and maintain cardiorespiratory endurance, it is important to know: (1) how to determine your target heart rate range, (2) how to measure your heart rate, (3) what type of exercises, (4) what types of training methods to use, and (5) what are the effective exercise strategies.

TABLE 5.1

*Formula and Example for Calculating the Target Heart Rate Range
(Example will use a 20-year-old exerciser.)*

Formula for Calculations	Example	Space to Figure Your Target Range
Step 1. Take 220 and subtract your age. This gives your estimated maximum heart rate.	200 − 20 ─────── = 200 beats per minute (bpm) is the estimated maximum heart rate	
Step 2. Take 200 and multiply by .60 to determine the lower limit of target heart rate range.	200 × .60 ─────── = 120 bpm is the lower limit of target heart rate range	
Step 3. Take 200 and multiply by .90 to determine the upper limit of target heart rate range.	200 × .90 ─────── = 180 bpm is the upper limit of target heart rate range	

* 120 to 180 bpm is the target heart rate
range for this 20-year-old exerciser.

Note: 60–70% of Maximum Heart Rate: Beginner exercisers should strive for
70–80% of Maximum Heart Rate: Intermediate exercisers should strive for
80–90% of Maximum Heart Rate: Advanced athletes should strive for

Source: Guidelines for Exercise Testing and Prescription *(5th ed.), American College of Sports Medicine, 1995.*

How to Determine Your Estimated Target Heart Rate Range

Your target heart rate range is the number of beats per minute (bpm) your heart should beat during exercise. It is one of the best indicators to determine if you are exercising at the right intensity. When you exercise, your heart beats faster to meet the demand for more blood and oxygen by your working muscles. The more intense the exercise, the faster your heart will beat. Therefore, monitoring your heart rate during exercise is a excellent way to monitor your exercise intensity.

For exercisers, there is a range of exercise intensities that is described as safe and effective for promoting cardiovascular benefits. Your estimated target heart rate range can be determined by calculating a lower and upper limit. During exercise, raise your heart rate at least to the lower limit but not above the upper limit. If you are just beginning a fitness program, you should probably aim for the lower limit and pick up the intensity as you become more comfortable with exercise. If you are more fit, you should strive for the middle of the range. If you have a good base and are in training for competitive events, you may want to aim for the upper limit.

These numbers serve only as guidelines and are recommended for individuals without any health problems. If you are taking medication that alters your heart rate, consult your physician for your recommended exercise intensity. Remember that your estimated target heart rate range is just that—an estimate. If you feel like you are exercising too hard, you probably are. Reduce your intensity and find a pace that works best for you.

Although there are other ways to calculate estimated target heart rate range, the method shown in table 5.1 is the easiest and safest for beginners. You can figure your estimated target heart rate range on the right side of this table.

How to Measure Your Heart Rate

To determine if you are exercising at the right intensity, it is important to know how to measure your heart rate. The two arteries used for counting pulse are the radial (palm side of your forearm on the thumb side of your wrist) and the carotid (on both sides of the Adam's apple). To count your pulse, place your index and middle fingertips over either the radial or carotid artery. Press gently to prevent cutting off the blood flow. Using the thumb is not ad-

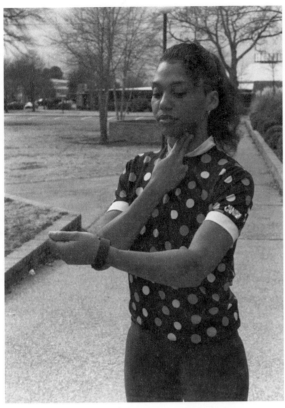
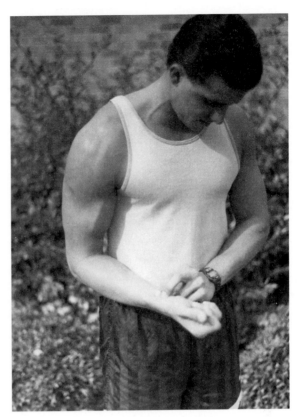

Use either the carotid artery or radial artery to count your pulse.

vised because it has its own strong pulse. Most exercisers use the carotid artery in the neck because it is easy to locate.

The most practical method is to measure your heart rate after the aerobic workout is completed. During the actual exercise would be the ideal time to measure your exercise heart rate. However, counting your pulse during exercise is difficult. Equipment like pulsemeters can be helpful to monitor your exercise heart rate, but most people do not have access to them. This is why it is more practical to wait until the workout has been completed.

For accurate results, it is important to measure your heart rate immediately after completing your workout. Your heart rate increases quickly during exercise and decreases just as quickly immediately after exercise. Waiting too long to measure your pulse after exercise and counting too long will result in incorrect readings. The key is to locate your heart rate quickly and count for a short time, beginning with zero.

Continue moving as you locate your pulse to prevent blood pooling. Then stop and count your heart rate for either six seconds, ten seconds, or fifteen seconds. To obtain your one-minute heart rate, perform the following functions: multiply by ten the number of beats you counted in the six-second period, multi-

ply by six the number of beats counted in the ten-second period, and multiply by four the number of beats counted in the fifteen-second period. Be accurate with your measurement—missing one or two beats could significantly distort your calculations.

Types of Effective Exercises

Aerobic and anaerobic are both effective methods to develop cardiorespiratory endurance. Aerobic exercises are, as mentioned earlier, activities in which the body is able to supply enough oxygen to the working muscles to sustain them for long periods of time. Because aerobic exercise is low to moderate in intensity and can be performed continuously, it is the most common type of exercise to develop cardiorespiratory fitness. By increasing intensity from moderate to high, you can quickly change your activity from aerobic to anaerobic. Swimming at a comfortable but brisk pace is aerobic; sprinting the last lap to finish your workout is anaerobic.

Anaerobic exercise is a short-term strenuous activity performed without an adequate oxygen supply. This type of exercise is performed at such a high rate of intensity that the body's demand for sufficient oxygen exceeds its ability to supply it. Because of its vigorous nature, anaerobic exercise is usually reserved for competitive athletes.

TABLE 5.2

Effective Exercise Strategies for Cardiorespiratory Endurance

Mode: Any activity that is continuous, rhythmic, and uses the large muscle groups, e.g., running-jogging, walking-hiking, swimming, skating, bicycling, rowing, cross-country skiing, rope jumping, or various endurance game activities.

Frequency: 3 to 5 days per week.

Intensity: 60% to 90% of maximal heart rate. It should be noted that exercise of lower intensity may provide important health benefits and may result in increased fitness in some persons (e.g., those who were previously sedentary and had low fitness).

   A simple method to determine level of exertion is the "talk test." Intensity is too low if conversation can be maintained easily, whereas an inability to talk indicates the intensity is too high.

Time: 20 to 60 minutes of continuous aerobic activity. (20 to 30 minutes works well for most.) For those who are severely deconditioned, multiple sessions of short duration (about 10 minutes) may be necessary.

Rate of progression: In continuous exercise, this occurs by an increase in intensity, time, or some combination of the two. The most significant conditioning effects may be observed during the first six to eight weeks of the exercise program.

Source: Guidelines for Exercise Testing and Prescription *(5th ed.), American College of Sports Medicine, 1995.*

Types of Training Methods

Continuous

Continuous training refers to engaging in aerobic activities or sports where most of the large muscle groups are worked at low intensity. This type of training allows the activity to continue for a minimum of twenty to thirty minutes without stopping. Exercises performed continuously and rhythmically at low intensity are safer and more comfortable than high-intensity exercises. This is why the majority of participants choose aerobic exercises. However, overuse injuries to joints, ligaments, and muscles become possible when continuous movement is repeated for longer sessions. Cross-training or alternating exercises can prevent overuse injuries.

Interval

Interval training involves alternating an equal period of work with a period of rest. The intensity of the exercise may vary between 60 percent and 95 percent of maximum heart rate. The rest periods may be walking, jogging, or complete rest. For this type of training, the heart rate should not drop below 120 before the next work interval starts. Some runners like to sprint the straightaways on a track and walk the curves. Completing interval work sessions at high intensity places the participant at greater risk for injury and staleness. However, there are also advantages of interval training: It improves the body's ability to handle fatigue, it more closely resembles athletic events, and quality workouts can be achieved in less time.

Effective Exercise Strategies

The effective exercise strategies to develop cardiorespiratory endurance are highlighted in table 5.2.

HOW TO MEASURE CARDIORESPIRATORY ENDURANCE

Maximal oxygen uptake or VO_2max is the most precise method of evaluating cardiorespiratory endurance. VO_2max is defined as the greatest rate at which oxygen can be taken and used during exercise. To find out your VO_2max would require a laboratory and facilities not readily available for most people. However, there are several field tests that can be easily completed and will provide good estimates of your cardiorespiratory fitness level. The Step Test and Cooper's 1.5-Mile Test (see Activity 5B) are two examples. Table 5.3 shows the ratings for both tests.

SUMMARY

- Physical fitness experts usually consider cardiorespiratory endurance to be the most important component of health-related fitness. It has achieved its high status in the medical world because of its value in combating heart disease, strokes, high blood pressure, obesity, and stress. This component of fitness is also important to many types of work, play, and sports activities.
- Cardiorespiratory endurance involves the capacity to continue vigorous total body activity for a relatively long period of time. It is the ability of your heart, lungs, blood vessels, and blood to effectively supply oxygen and nutrients to the working muscles while removing waste products.
- The following characteristics are necessary to achieve cardiorespiratory endurance: a fit heart

TABLE 5.3

Ratings for the Step Test and 1.5-Mile Test

	Step Test (Heartbeats per Minute)		1.5-Mile Test (Time in Minutes)	
Ratings	*Men*	*Women*	*Men*	*Women*
Good	<79	<89	<12	<14
Fair	80–90	90–100	12–16	14–20
Low	91>	101>	16>	20>

Note: These standards have been designed for the 18- to 26-year-old age group. Younger and older populations may have more difficulty reaching the higher levels of achievement.

muscle, a fit blood vessel system, fit blood, and fit muscle tissue.

- When you participate in a cardiorespiratory fitness program with appropriate and sufficient frequency, intensity, and time (duration), your body will respond with numerous positive changes. Some of these include a larger, stronger, and more efficient heart muscle (especially in the left ventricle), healthier blood vessels, a decrease in resting heart rate, and an increase in mental benefits.
- To develop cardiorespiratory endurance, it is important to know how to determine your estimated target heart rate range, how to measure your heart rate, what type of exercises and training methods to use, and what are the effective exercise strategies.
- The two arteries used for counting pulse are the radial (palm side of your forearm on the thumb side of your wrist) and the carotid (on both sides of the Adam's apple).

- Your target heart rate range can be determined by calculating a lower limit and upper limit. To receive optimal value from your workout, raise your heart rate during exercise at least to the lower limit but not above the upper limit. Table 5.1 provides an example.
- Aerobic and anaerobic exercise are both effective methods to develop cardiorespiratory endurance.
- The two types of training are continuous and interval.
- Table 5.2 provides the effective exercise strategies to develop cardiorespiratory endurance.
- Maximal oxygen uptake or VO_2max is the most precise method of evaluating cardiorespiratory endurance. However, expensive equipment and a laboratory are required.

ACTIVITY   5A

MEASURING HEART RATE

Name _____   **To be submitted: Yes   No**

Date _____   **If yes, due date** _____

Class _____ Section _____   **Score** _____

PURPOSE
1. To practice counting your radial and carotid pulse.
2. To determine your target heart rate zone.
3. To participate in an exercise with the right amount of intensity to maintain your heart rate in the target zone.

DIRECTIONS
1. Practice counting your pulse for 6, 10, and 15 seconds by using the carotid and radial arteries (see page 58). To determine your heart rate in beats per minute, add a zero to the number of beats in 6 seconds. For 10 and 15 seconds, count the number of beats and multiply by six and four, respectively.
2. Using table 5.1 on page 58, figure out your own target heart rate range. Have a partner or your instructor check your work.
3. Strive to raise your heart rate into the target range by participating in a physical activity for 20 minutes. Your instructor may allow you to choose your own exercise, or he or she may have chosen a class exercise (jogging, fitness wal..ing, etc.). After 10 minutes of exercising, check heart rate. After 20 minutes, recheck heart rate.
4. Answer questions in the Results section.

RESULTS
1. What were your heart rate measurements?

				Radial	Carotid
Six-second count	×	10	=	_____	_____
Ten-second count	×	6	=	_____	_____
Fifteen-second count	×	4	=	_____	_____

2. What is your target heart rate range?

   Lower limit _____ Upper limit _____

3. What was your heart rate after the 10-minute exercise period? _____

   What was your heart rate after the 20-minute exercise period? _____

   Were you able to maintain the desired intensity for your target range?   Yes   No

ACTIVITY   5B

MEASURING CARDIORESPIRATORY ENDURANCE

Name _____   *To be submitted:* Yes   No

Date _____   *If yes, due date* _____

Class _____ Section _____   Score _____

PURPOSE
To evaluate your cardiorespiratory endurance with a 3-minute step test and a 1.5-mile run.

DIRECTIONS

STEP TEST
1. Warm up before taking the step test and cool down after finishing it.
2. For 3 minutes, continuously step up and down on an 8-inch bench at a 24-steps-per-minute rate. One cycle consists of "up with the left foot, up with the right foot, down with the left foot, down with the right foot."
3. Immediately after the 3 minutes of stepping, sit down and rest for 1 minute.
4. After the 1-minute rest, complete a 30-second count pulse.
5. Multiply the number of heartbeats during the 30-second period by two for your score.
6. Refer to table 5.3 on page 00 to rate your score and record in the Results section.

1.5-MILE TEST
1. Make sure you are medically ready for this endurance test.
2. Warm up before taking the 1.5-mile test and cool down after finishing it.
3. Begin the test and cover the distance in the fastest time possible. You may want to start out jogging and resort to fast walking if you get tired. If any unusual symptoms arise during the test, stop and retake the test after six weeks of aerobic exercise.
4. Record the time it took to complete the 1.5-mile test.
5. Refer to table 5.3 on page 61 to rate your score and record in the Results section.

RESULTS
1. Record the information from taking one or both cardiorespiratory endurance tests in the space provided.

   Step Test

   Beats per 30 seconds _____ × 2 = _____ Rating _____

   1.5 Mile Test

   Time to complete 1.5 mile test _____ Rating _____

2. If you took both tests, were the results similar?   Yes   No   Explain.

3. What did your results tell you?

4. Are you satisfied with your cardiorespiratory endurance?   Yes   No   Explain.

5. What fitness activities do you enjoy that would either improve or maintain your level of cardiorespiratory endurance?

STRATEGIES FOR STRENGTH AND MUSCULAR ENDURANCE

Possessing strength and muscular endurance are two essential qualities to attain a high level of fitness and health!

LEARNING OBJECTIVES

- Define strength and muscular endurance.
- Identify several possible benefits of weight training.
- Describe the training effects of a weight-training program.
- Identify and briefly describe the two methods for improving strength and muscular endurance.
- Compare the advantages and disadvantages of free weights versus machines.
- Discuss several strategies for weight training.
- Evaluate your strength and muscular endurance.

LIFESTYLE QUESTIONS

- Have you ever performed calisthenics such as push-ups, sit-ups, jumping jacks, and so on?
- Have you ever participated in a weight-training program, using free weights or machine weights?
- Do you know a friend or family member who participates in weight training or calisthenics?
- Are you satisfied with the level of strength you possess?
- Are you satisfied with the level of muscular endurance you possess?
- If you are not currently involved in a weight-training program, would you consider participating in one?

INTRODUCTION

Strength and muscular endurance are two important health-related components of physical fitness. **Strength** is defined as the maximum amount of force a muscle or a group of muscles can exert at one time. It is a necessary component to improve your fitness and overall health. Strength is also an important fitness component in almost every athletic performance. Of equal importance, weight training to improve strength is now a socially acceptable and respectable activity for both men and women.

Muscular endurance is defined as the ability of the muscles to perform contractions repeatedly over a period of time or to hold a position for an extended period of time. Muscular endurance is also an essential component to improve your fitness and overall health. For most activities, strength and muscular en-

durance complement each other. For example, it's not enough to have adequate strength for lifting a shovelful of dirt—you have to be able to keep shoveling until the dirt pile is gone.

BENEFITS OF MODERATE WEIGHT TRAINING

By engaging in a moderate weight-training program, you can receive numerous health and fitness benefits (see table 6.1).

ADAPTATIONS TO TRAINING

When you engage in regular exercise of moderate-to-high intensity, the different systems of your body will

TABLE 6.1

Benefits of Moderate Weight Training

1. Leads to a trimmer, firmer body
2. Increases self-confidence
3. Aids in weight control (adding a pound of muscle tissue to a person's body weight will increase the basal metabolic rate [BMR] by 35 calories per day)
4. Elevates mood
5. Improves posture
6. Increases energy
7. Leads to fewer injuries in other activities
8. Prevents frequent back trouble
9. Helps strengthen bones and prevent osteoporosis
10. Helps the older adult feel and perform better
11. Improves ability to do everyday chores
12. May lower blood pressure and LDL (bad) cholesterol
13. May stabilize blood sugar levels in diabetics

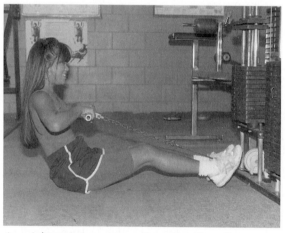

A weight-training program has many benefits.

respond by making **physiological adaptations** or changes. If these adaptations are significant, they are called **training effects.** The extent of the training effect will depend on the type, frequency, intensity, and time (duration) of your exercise. For example, aerobic activities like jogging will improve your cardiorespiratory fitness but do little for improving your upper body strength.

The rate of increase using progressive resistance training will depend on the type and emphasis of **training.** Progressive resistance training will increase both strength and muscular endurance simultaneously. However, what improves the most depends on your training. Using a **resistance** or weight that is so heavy only a few **repetitions** (one rep is performing the exercise one time) can be completed will produce a greater increase in strength than in muscular endurance. Using a resistance that is light enough in weight to complete at least fifteen repetitions will produce a greater increase in muscular endurance than in strength (see fig. 6.1). Regardless of the resistance or weight you use, strength and muscular endurance cannot be increased or decreased without affecting each other.

Hypertrophy, or an increase in muscle size, is the most visible adaptation to strength training. It is generally believed that training produces an increase in the size of each fiber (hypertrophy) involved rather than an increase in the number of fibers (**hyperplasia**). Some investigators have reported heavy resistance training causes fibers to split. However, there is no substantial evidence of real cell division (**mitosis**) resulting from training. **Atrophy,** or a decrease in muscle size, results when there is a lack of stimulation of the muscle. If you stop your weight-training program, you can expect your trained muscles to atrophy. Also, atrophy will occur if your muscles become immobilized by complete bed rest, placing a limb in a cast, or nerve failure. See figure 6.2 for a diagram of the muscles of the body.

Along with the other health-related components of fitness, a high fitness level of strength and muscular endurance are temporary qualities. You receive the benefits as long as you stay with your weight-training program and lose them when you stop doing it. One or two weight-training and aerobic workouts per week will maintain strength and muscular endurance at a relatively constant level.

Muscle strength can be gained without a significant increase in muscle size. Individuals past sixty years of age apparently have little capacity for increasing muscle size. Nonetheless, they can exhibit an increase in strength when engaged in regular resistance exercises for six to eight weeks. This gain in strength is attributed to a greater than usual activation of muscle fibers by the central nervous system. It is also believed that increased neural efficiency is the reason why a young person makes early gains in strength during the first three to four weeks.

Women who perform the same training program as men experience similar gains in strength but not in size. The greater increase in the size of the muscle cells for men is attributed to testosterone, a

FIGURE 6.1

Relationship between Strength and Endurance Training

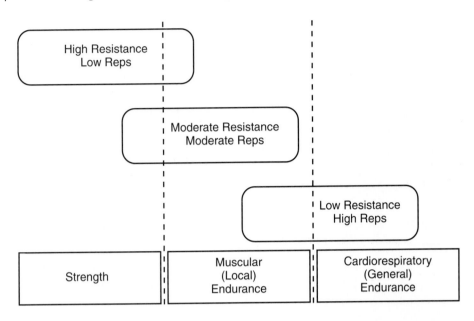

male hormone. The strength gains of women compare favorably with men when lean body weight is used. Even closer results are exhibited when men and women are compared by the strength of the large muscles of the lower body.

The number of muscle fibers and their arrangements influence adaptations. Two people, regardless of age or sex, can perform the same training program and differ significantly in their physical adaptations. **Mesomorphs** (muscular build) are born with more muscle tissue than **endomorphs** (medium build) and **ectomorphs** (lean build). In addition, men usually have more muscle tissue than women, which at least partially accounts for more rapid gains of strength.

METHODS TO DEVELOP STRENGTH AND MUSCULAR ENDURANCE

Isometric and dynamic training are the two methods for developing strength and muscular endurance.

Isometric

Isometrics involves a contraction without movement or a force applied against an immovable object. The muscles do not change length in isometrics like they will in dynamic exercises. Pushing your hands against each other is an example of an isometric contraction. To develop strength using isometric training, hold a maximum or near maximum contraction for six to ten seconds several times a day. The following considerations should be kept in mind when using static or isometric weight training:

1. It does not increase strength through the entire range of motion—only at the joint angles at which the contraction takes place.
2. It can be dangerous for older people to perform, especially those with high blood pressure because the breath is usually held during the isometric contraction.
3. It does not increase the size of the muscle.

Dynamic

By far the more popular of the two, the dynamic method includes isotonic and isokinetic types of weight training. Isotonic training involves concentric and eccentric contractions. In **concentric contractions,** the muscle fibers shorten. In **eccentric contractions,** the muscle fibers lengthen. Calisthenics such as push-ups and pull-ups are considered isotonic because the muscles change length by shortening and lengthening. However, weight training is considered the most effective method for improving strength and muscular endurance.

FIGURE 6.2

The Major Muscle Groups

THE MAJOR MUSCLE GROUPS

Trapezius (Traps)

Sternocleido-mastoid

Deltoid (Delts)

Pectoralis Major (Pecs)

Brachialis

Biceps Brachii (Biceps)

Brachioradialis

Psoas (Hip Flexor) (Under Abdominals) Not Visible

Gracilis

(a) Rectus Femoris

(a) Vastus Medialis

Gastrocnemius

Soleus (Calf)

Latissimus Dorsi (Lats)

External Oblique (Obliques)

Rectus Abdominis (Abs)

Sartorius

Adductor Longus

(a) Vastus Lateralis

Margulies/Waldrop

Brachialis

Sternocleidomastoid

Trapezius (Traps)

Deltoid (Delts)

Triceps Brachii (Triceps)

Brachio-radialis

(b) Biceps Femoris

(b) Semitendinosus

(b) Semimembranosus

Gastrocnemius (Calf)

Achilles Tendon

Rhomboideus (Rhomboids)

Latissimus Dorsi (Lats)

External Oblique (Obliques)

Gluteus Maximus (Gluts)

Adductor Magnus

Gracilis

Sartorius

Soleus (Calf)

Margulies/Waldrop

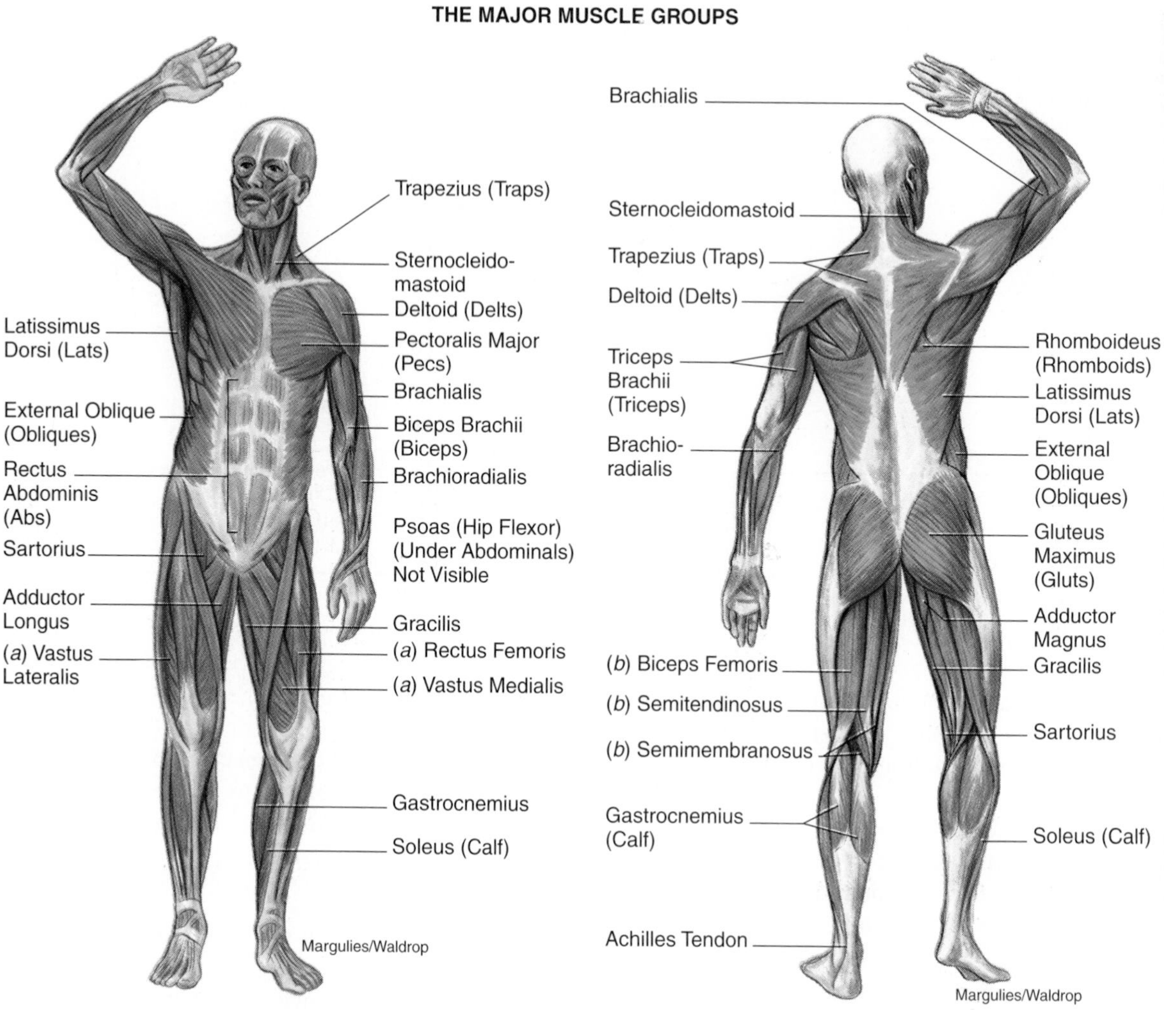

(a) Quadriceps (Quads) include the four muscles identified by the letter (a) and the vastus intermedius (under the Rectus Femoris) not visible.

(b) Hamstrings (Hams) are the three muscles identified by the letter (b).

From Kent M. Van De Graaff and Stuart Ira Fox, Concepts of Human Anatomy and Physiology, 3d ed. Copyright © 1992 Wm. C. Brown Communications, Inc., Dubuque, Iowa. All Rights Reserved. Reprinted by permission.

The principle of progressive overload can be more easily applied in weight training than in calisthenics. Weight training allows the amount of resistance to be changed. For your muscles to become stronger, they must be regularly challenged beyond what they normally do. If the overload is appropriate, your muscle(s) will be able to respond by adapting and increasing in strength. If the overload is too great, the result could be extreme soreness or even injury.

Dr. DeLorme in the 1940s was the first to organize weight lifting into the traditional three sets of ten repetitions. The ten-repetition maximum

(10–RM) was first determined by finding the greatest resistance that can be lifted ten times but not more than ten consecutive times. The traditional DeLorme system:

First set: 10 repetitions at 50% of the 10–RM set
Second set: 10 repetitions at 75% of the 10–RM set
Third set: 10 repetitions at 100% of the 10–RM set

When the individual was able to perform more than ten repetitions during the third set, a new 10–RM would be established and more weight added.

With some variations, strength programs have followed the DeLorme system for more than fifty

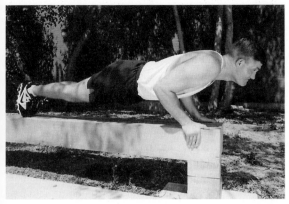

Holding a push-up at midpoint is an example of an isometric contraction.

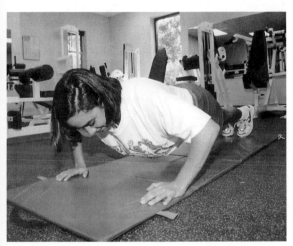

Performing a normal push-up is an example of a dynamic contraction.

years. For general fitness, three **sets** (the number of reps performed without rest) is the usual number that is completed. With advanced strength training, the average number of sets is between four to six. Bodybuilders may perform as many as eight sets in their programs. Approximately ten **reps** (i.e., ten arm curls) are usually completed in each set. In advanced strength training, weight lifters perform four to six reps per set whereas bodybuilders may complete as many as twenty reps per set.

Determining the amount of resistance (how much weight to use) may be based on the De-Lorme 10–RM or a single maximum repetition, 1–RM. Training programs for both fitness and body-building compute to 75 percent of the participant's 10–RM or 1–RM. Advanced strength training may use 75 to 100 percent of the participant's 1–RM. Although many bodybuilders may rest only thirty seconds between sets, most programs suggest taking a one- to two-minute rest. Because advanced strength-

training persons exercise at close to their 1–RM, they may require up to five or six minutes of rest between each exhaustive set.

The frequency of workouts recommended per week is still three, with a day of rest (recovery) between each session. Utilizing variations of split routines, advanced strength programs and bodybuilding allow daily workouts. See table 6.2 for a summary of effective exercise strategies for strength training using isotonic and isokinetic methods.

Isokinetic contractions incorporate the positive aspects of isometric and isotonic contractions while leaving out their weaknesses. In isokinetic contractions, the speed is constant regardless of the force applied, and 100 percent of maximum contraction is permitted through an entire range of motion. In isotonic contraction, the resistance is constant and a full range of motion is permitted. However, a maximum contraction will only take place at the weakest point during the range of motion. In isometric contraction, the range of motion is constant and a maximum contraction is allowed only at the specific joint angle.

Free weights or weight machines—which type is best? Both types are excellent, with each having advantages and disadvantages (see table 6.3). Free weights include barbells and dumbbells, along with homemade weights such as plastic bottles filled with sand or water. Weight machines include Marcy, Hydra-Gym, Dynacam, Universal, Nautilus, and Mini Gym. If you can, experiment with both free weights and weight machines to determine which is the preferred method for you.

STRATEGIES FOR WEIGHT TRAINING

Get some expert advice before starting a weight-training program. To learn the correct techniques, consult with your instructor, sign up for a weight-training class, or join a health club.

Warm up and cool down properly. This will better prepare your muscles and joints for the workout. It can also help prevent or reduce muscle soreness and injury.

Know your goals. To train for strength, lift heavy weights a few times. To train for muscular endurance, lift light weights many times.

Exercise all major parts of the body—arms, legs, chest, stomach, and back. Exercise the muscles on both sides of each limb. For example, if the muscles located on the front of the upper arms are exercised (by curls or chin-ups), the muscles on the

TABLE 6.2

Effective Exercise Strategies for Strength Training (Isotonic and Isokinetic)

	General Fitness	**Advanced Strength**	**Bodybuilders**
Sets	3	3–6	4–8
Reps	10	4–6	12–20
Rest	1–2 min. rest between sets	30 sec. up to 5–6 min.	30 sec. up to 5–6 min.
Amount of Resistance	75% of max. rep.	75–100% of max. rep.	75–100% max. rep.
Frequency	3 days a week	Daily using different muscles	Daily using different muscles

TABLE 6.3

Free Weights Versus Machines

Free Weights

Advantages	*Disadvantages*
1. No restricted motion and can move in many different directions.	1. Create more possibility of injury.
2. Truer to real-life situation, so skills transfer to daily life.	2. Require spotters for safety.
3. Less expensive.	3. Take additional time to change weights.
4. Very convenient if located at your residence.	4. The different parts can get lost or stolen.
5. Unlimited number of exercises available.	5. Require more balance and coordination so more muscles are needed for stabilization.

Weight Machines

Advantages	*Disadvantages*
1. Other body parts are stabilized, so easier to isolate a muscle or muscle group.	1. Restricted to range and angle of movement permitted by the machine.
2. Safer because weight is not able to fall on you.	2. Expensive to afford on your own.
3. No spotters needed.	3. The controlled path of weight is not true to real life.
4. Easy and quick to change weights.	4. May have to wait in line to use the machine.

back of the upper arms should also be exercised (by push-ups or bench presses).

Exercise each muscle group through the joint's full range of motion. You will receive the most benefit from your weight-training program by performing the techniques correctly.

Start off with a weight you can comfortably lift. As you get stronger, gradually add more weight and/or increase the number of repetitions. (See table 6.4 for guidelines.)

Do not hold your breath while performing a lift. A good rule of thumb is exhale as you lift the weight and inhale as you let it down.

Listen to your body. Feeling pain is a warning sign that you should stop and seek help.

Consider joining a certified health club. Nice equipment is usually available, staff members can provide instruction, and club members can provide inspiration.

Consider using free weights or weight machines at home. Having weights at your convenience is an important consideration for sticking with a weight-training program.

Wait at least forty-eight hours before exercising the same body parts again. Muscles grow by recuperating after the workout. The same muscles exercised every day will not have time to recuperate and fitness gains will be diminished.

Enjoy weight training. Although weight training can be challenging, it can be rewarding and fun, too.

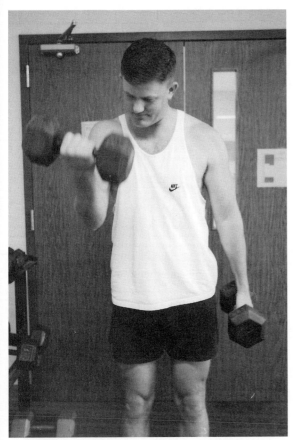

Free weights

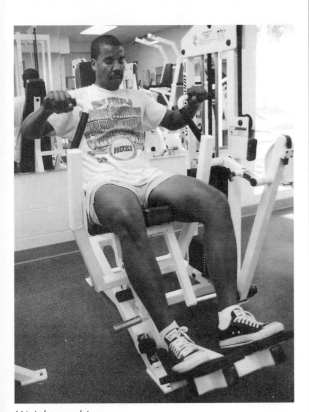

Weight machine

TABLE 6.4

Effective Exercise Strategies for Dynamic Muscular Endurance Training

Frequency:	3 to 4 days per week
Intensity:	20% to 70% of the maximum resistance you can lift or simply select a light weight you can lift comfortably
Time:	1 to 5 sets of 9 to 25 reps for each exercise—rest 30 seconds between sets

Note: Beginners are encouraged to start out at the minimum guidelines and progress slowly.

Perceiving weight training as a positive experience can help keep you motivated for a lifetime.

HOW TO EVALUATE STRENGTH AND MUSCULAR ENDURANCE

There are many ways to measure strength and muscular endurance. When available, dynamometers and cable tensiometers can be used to measure strength and muscular endurance isometrically. Dynamic strength can be tested by performing a one-repetition maximum contraction using weights as the resistance. To do this, you can use a bench or leg press, or a pull-up with weights attached to yourself.

Testing accurately is important for measuring strength and muscular endurance. Since strength is the force of a single maximum contraction, if more than one repetition is completed in an assessment, the validity of the test is reduced. For example, a one-minute sit-up test will evaluate muscular endurance more than it will evaluate strength. A more accurate test of abdominal strength is to place sufficient weight on your chest that would restrict you from doing more than one sit-up.

Strength and Muscular Endurance Tests

This section offers four different strength and muscular endurance tests, which are included in Activity 6A. Follow directions carefully for each test. Ratings for the tests are given in table 6.5.

Test 1: Grip Strength

Hold and squeeze the dynamometer as hard as possible using only one hand. You can straighten or bend the arm, but you are not allowed to touch your body with your hand, elbow, or arm. The score is the best of two trials recorded in pounds.

TABLE 6.5

Ratings for Strength and Muscular Endurance Tests

Ratings	Grip Strength	Sit-Ups	Push-Ups	
	Men	Women	Men	Women
Good	136>	81>	41>	36>
Fair	100–135	55–80	30–40	25–35
Low	<99	<54	<29	<24

Ratings	Modified Push-Ups	Pull-Ups	Bent-Arm Hang
Good	31>	13>	21> sec.
Fair	20–30	8–12	15–20 sec.
Low	<19	<7	<14 sec.

Note: These standards have been designed for the 18- to 26-year-old age group. Younger and older populations may have more difficulty reaching the higher levels of achievement.

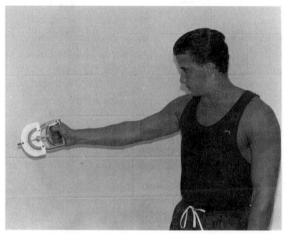

Grip strength

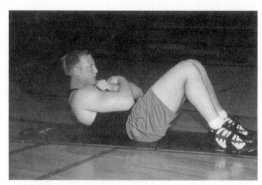

Performing a proper sit-up

Test 2: Sit-Ups

Perform as many modified sit-ups as possible in sixty seconds. The starting position is lay flat on the mat. Keep knees bent and feet flat on the mat. Contract abdominals by raising shoulder blades 1-2 inches off the mat while keeping lower back intact with the mat. Return to starting position.

Test 3: Push-Ups and Modified Push-Ups

Push-ups: Lie in a prone position, supporting your body on your hands and toes with elbows fully extended. *Modified push-ups:* Do the same, except support your body on hands and knees. With both types, keep your knees together, place your hands about shoulder-width apart, hold your back straight, and keep your head down with eyes looking slightly ahead.

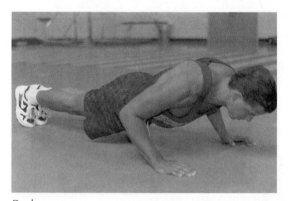

Push-up

Keeping the body rigid, bend your elbows until your chest touches the floor, then return to the starting position. Partner counts how many times in one minute you return to an upright position.

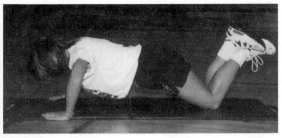

Modified push-up

Test 4: Pull-Ups and Bent-Arm Hang

Pull-ups: Hang from a bar with your arms fully extended. Your hands should be a little farther than shoulder-width apart with palms facing away from you. Without kicking, swaying, or jerking, raise your body upward until your chin is above the bar. Then lower yourself to the starting position with arms fully extended. Your score is the number of pull-ups you can do in one minute.

    Bent-arm hang: With your hands placed on the bar a little farther than shoulder-width apart and your palms facing you, place your chin above the bar but not touching it. You may need a chair to do this. Hold your chin over the bar for as long as possible. Have a partner or your instructor count the number of seconds you can keep your chin above the bar without touching it. Maximum score is sixty.

STRENGTH AND MUSCULAR ENDURANCE PROGRAMS

Program 1: Weight Training Machine Exercises

Here is an example of a weight training program using Body Masters Equipment.

    For directions to use this and other types of weight equipment, check with your instructor. You can also refer to the instructor's manual for the equipment.

1. Leg Press
   Muscles trained: Quadriceps, Hamstrings, Gluteus
2. Leg Extensions
   Muscles trained: Quadriceps
3. Hamstring Curl
   Muscles trained: Hamstrings
4. Heel Raises
   Muscles trained: Calf
5. Vertical Chest Press
   Muscles trained: Pectorals, Deltoids, Triceps
6. Lat Pull-Down
   Muscles trained: Latissmus ("lats"), biceps, and pectorals

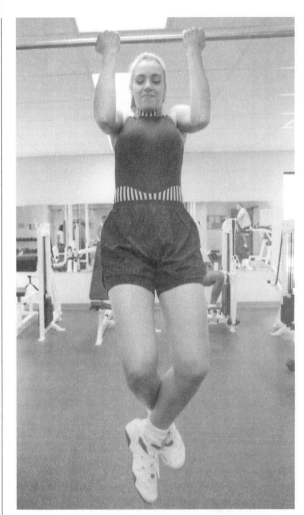

A pull-up

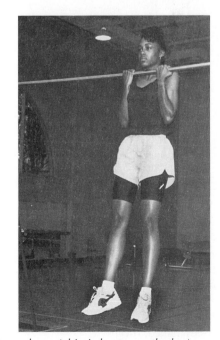

Bent-arm hang (chin is kept over the bar)

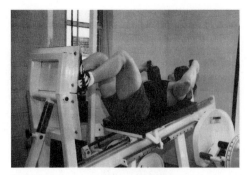

Leg press

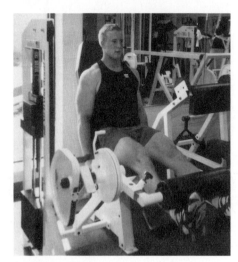

Leg Extensions

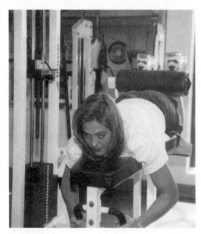

Hamstring curl

7. Seated Row
    Muscles trained: Upper arms and shoulders, lats, trapezius, deltoids
8. Shoulder Press
    Muscles trained: Deltoids, Triceps
9. Bicep Curl
    Muscles trained: Biceps

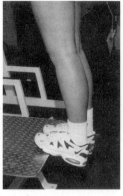

*Heel raises
(starting position)*

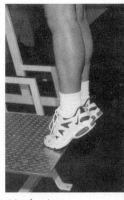

*Heel raises
(ending position)*

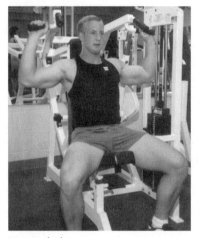

Vertical chest press

10. Tricep Press
    Muscles trained: Triceps
11. Dips
    Muscles Trained: Pectorals, Triceps
12. Pull-Ups
    Muscles trained: Arms and Shoulder muscles, biceps, deltoids, forearms, pect
13. Hip Flexors
    Muscles trained: Hip Flexors, Lower Abdominals

Program 2: Building Strength and Muscular Endurance through Calisthenics

Perform as many repetitions as you can without straining.

1. **Push-Ups**
    Muscles: Arm, shoulder, and chest
    Starting Position: Lie in a prone position, supporting your body on your hands and toes with elbows fully extended. With your knees together and back straight, place your hands shoulder-width apart and head down with eyes looking slightly ahead.

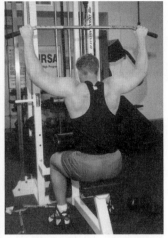

Lat pull-down (starting position)

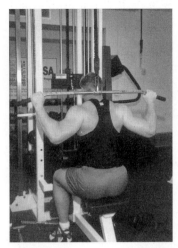

Lat pull-down (with variation)

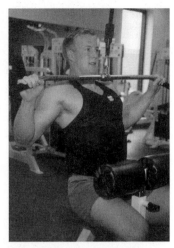

Lat pull-down (ending position)

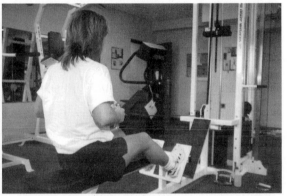

Seated row

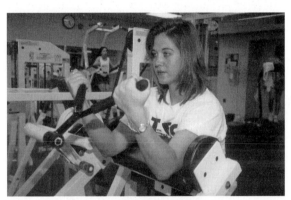

Bicep curl

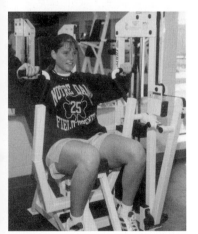

Shoulder press

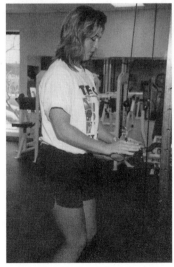

Triceps press

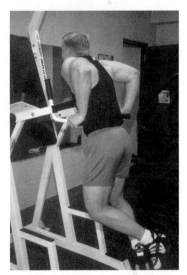

Dips

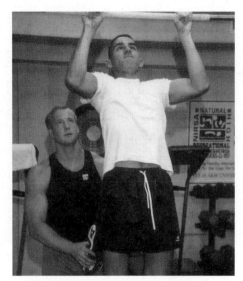

Pull-ups

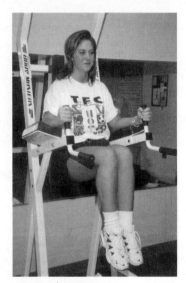

Hip flexors

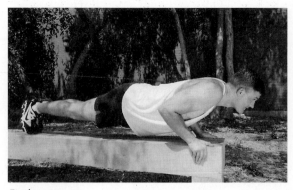

Push-up

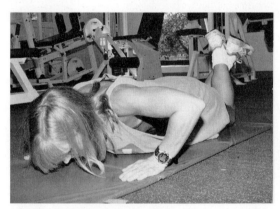

Modified push-up

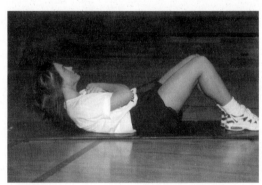

Curl-up

Movement: Keeping the body rigid, bend elbows until the chest touches the floor, then return to starting position. Repeat.

2. **Modified Push-Ups** (For those who are not able to perform a regular push-up)

For this sh-up, follow the recommendations for the re ular push-up except place your weight on your knees instead of your toes.

3. **Curl-Ups**

Muscles: Upper stomach

Starting Position: Lie on your back with your legs bent or extended. Raise your feet off the floor slightly, keeping your legs parallel to the floor. Hold your arms across your chest or bring your palms to your ears. (For easier curl-ups, place hands at the side of your body.)

Movement: Curl up until your shoulder blades leave the floor. Then roll down to the starting position. Repeat.

4. **Reverse Curls**

Muscles: Lower stomach

Starting Position: Lie on your back with your knees bent. Place your feet flat on the floor and arms at sides.

Movement: Lift your knees to your chest and raise your hips off the floor. Do not let your knees go past your shoulders. Return to the starting position and repeat.

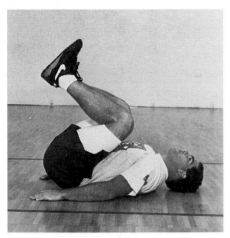
The reverse curl

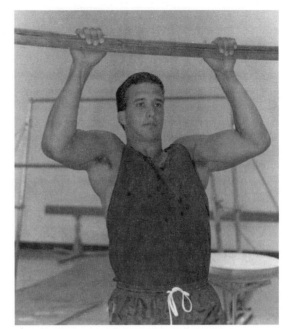
The pull-up

5. **Pull-Ups**
   Muscles: Arm and shoulder
   Starting Position: Hang from a bar with your arms fully extended. Your hands should be a little farther than shoulder-width apart with palms facing away from you.
   Movement: Without kicking, swaying, or jerking, raise your body upward until your chin is above the bar. Then lower yourself to the starting position with arms fully extended. Repeat.

6. **Modified Pull-Ups** (For those unable to perform a pull-up)
   Muscles: Arm and shoulder
   Starting Position: With your palms facing you and hands placed shoulder-width apart, hang from a low bar. Place your feet in front of the bar with your heels touching the floor. Keep your body rigid.
   Movement: Pull up, keeping your body straight. Touch your chest to the bar and then lower yourself to the starting position. Repeat.

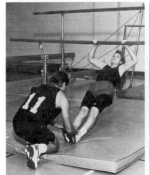 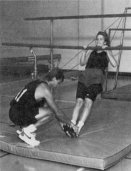
The modified pull-up (starting position)
The modified pull-up (finish position)

7. **Upper Back Lift**
   Muscles: Upper back
   Starting Position: Lie in the prone position with your arms held behind your head. Keep your hips and toes secured to the floor.
   Movement: Lift your upper body up as far as possible and hold for two seconds. Return and repeat.

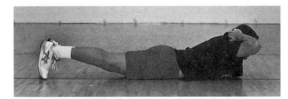
The upper back lift

8. **Lower Back Lift**
   Muscles: Lower back
   Starting Position: Lie in the prone position with your arms placed at your sides and your chin touching the floor.
   Movement: Alternate raising one leg slowly up and down.

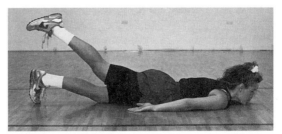
The lower back lift

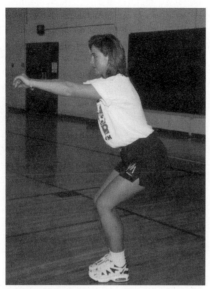

Half-squat

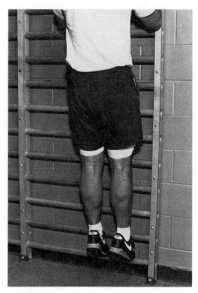

Heel raise

9. **Half-Squats**
   Muscles: Leg
   Starting Position: Stand erect with feet together and arms at your sides.
   Movement: Keeping your back straight, bend at the knee until calf and thigh muscle form about a ninety-degree angle. Do not go past the ninety-degree angle. Return to starting position and repeat.

10. **Heel Raise**
    Muscles: Calf
    Starting Position: Stand with the toes on a two-by-four or lower rung of a stall bar. Hold on to a support with your hands.
    Movement: Raise up on your toes as far as possible and hold for several seconds. Lower your heels as far as possible. Repeat.

SUMMARY

- Strength and muscular endurance are two important health-related components of physical fitness.
- Strength is defined as the maximum amount of force a muscle or a group of muscles can exert at one time.
- Muscular endurance is defined as the ability of the muscles to perform contractions repeatedly over a period of time or to hold a position for an extended period of time.
- For most activities, strength and muscular endurance complement each other. It's not enough to have adequate strength for lifting a shovelful of dirt—you have to be able to keep shoveling until the dirt pile is gone.

- By engaging in a moderate weight-training program, you can receive numerous health and fitness benefits (see table 6.1).
- When you engage in regular exercise of moderate-to-high intensity, the different systems of your body will respond by making physiological adaptations or changes. If these adaptations are significant, they are called training effects.
- The extent of the training effect will depend on the type, frequency, intensity, and time (duration) of your exercise.
- Isometric and dynamic training are the two methods for developing strength and muscular endurance.
- Isometrics involves a contraction without movement or a force applied against an immovable object. The muscles do not change length in isometrics like they will in dynamic exercises.
- The dynamic includes isotonic and isokinetic types of weight training. Isotonic training involves concentric and eccentric contractions. In concentric contractions, the muscle fibers shorten. In eccentric contractions, the muscle fibers lengthen.
- Weight training is considered the most effective method for improving strength and muscular endurance.
- Both free weights and weight machines are excellent for weight training. Each has its advantages and disadvantages (see table 6.3).
- There are many strategies to follow for a weight-training program.

A C T I V I T Y   **6A**

MEASURING STRENGTH AND MUSCULAR ENDURANCE

Name _____   **To be submitted: Yes   No**

Date _____   **If yes, due date** _____

Class _____   **Section** _____   **Score** _____

PURPOSE

1. To evaluate your grip strength using a hand dynamometer.

2. To evaluate the muscular endurance of your arms, shoulders, and chest by performing push-ups and pull-ups or modified push-ups and the bent-arm hang.

3. To evaluate the muscular endurance of your abdomen by performing sit-ups.

DIRECTIONS

1. Warm up properly before performing the tests.

2. Select a partner to assist you in performing and recording the activities.

3. Follow the exact instructions and perform each activity as described on pages 73 to 75.

4. Refer to table 6.5 on page 74 to rate your scores and record in the Results section.

5. Answer the questions in the Results section.

RESULTS

1. What were your strength and muscular endurance scores and ratings for the four tests?

	Scores	Ratings
Test 1: Grip Strength	_____	_____
Test 2: Sit-ups	_____	_____
Test 3: Push-Ups/Modified Push-Ups	_____	_____
Test 4: Pull-Ups/Bent-Arm Hang	_____	_____

2. How would you evaluate your current levels of strength and muscular endurance?

3. Do you plan to improve your levels of strength and muscular endurance?   Yes   No   If yes, what exercises will you use?

ACTIVITY   6B
PERFORMING A STRENGTH AND MUSCULAR ENDURANCE PROGRAM

Name _____   To be submitted: Yes   No

Date _____   If yes, due date _____

Class _____   Section _____   Score _____

PURPOSE
1. To provide some sample exercises that can be used to develop mild strength and muscular endurance.
2. To provide you an opportunity to experience a lifetime mild strength and muscular endurance program.

DIRECTIONS
1. First, warm up your muscles properly with a light aerobic workout and stretching.
2. Select one or both of the strength-training programs outlined on pages 75 to 80.
3. For the weight-machine program, perform five to ten repetitions using light weights.
4. For the calisthenics program, complete as many repetitions as possible without straining.

RESULTS
1. Which program(s) did you choose? Did you enjoy performing the strength and muscular endurance exercises?   Yes   No

2. Do you plan to include strength and muscular endurance exercises as part of your total fitness program?
   Yes   No   Explain.

CHAPTER 7

STRATEGIES FOR FLEXIBILITY

Make stretching a daily habit and especially include it as part of your physical fitness program!

INTRODUCTION

To have total fitness, you need to have at least adequate levels of flexibility. A goal for most of us is to have increased flexibility through stretching exercises.

CONSIDERATIONS FOR FLEXIBILITY

Being flexible has many advantages. Adequate range of motion can improve your athletic performance, reduce your soreness and injury to muscles and connective tissue, enable your body to move more and efficiently and gracefully. A daily stretching program that maintains an adequate level of flexibility can also lead to higher quality of life.

Being inflexible has disadvantages. Most injuries to muscle and connective tissue are primarily due to a lack of strength and flexibility. Muscles are more likely to be pulled or torn when they are tight and weak. An example of the relationship between strength and flexibility is low back pain—the number one health complaint heard by orthopedic surgeons and the number two complaint registered by internists. The troublesome, long-term condition of low back pain can often be prevented or improved by stretching the hip flexors and lower back muscles while strengthening the abdominal muscles.

Limitations to flexibility are determined by joint structure and the soft tissue around the joint. Most joints are influenced, to some extent, by the shape of their bones. The soft tissue around a joint includes muscle, connective tissue (fascial sheaths, tendons, ligaments, joint capsules), and skin. Research indicates the three most influential factors limiting range of motion are (1) muscles and their fascial sheaths, (2) the joint capsule, and (3) tendons.

Flexibility is specific to each joint. It is incorrect to talk about general flexibility. Among individuals, there can be differences in flexibility when comparing the same joint. In each person, the range of motion of all the joints can vary. Flexibility is specific to each

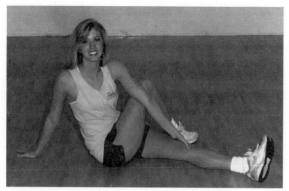

A stretching program can improve the quality of your life.

FIGURE 7.1
Balanced muscle strength and length permit good postural alignment.

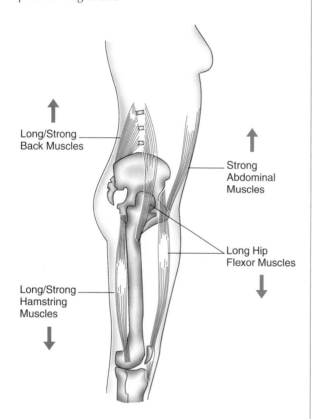

Long/Strong Back Muscles

Strong Abdominal Muscles

Long Hip Flexor Muscles

Long/Strong Hamstring Muscles

FIGURE 7.2
The Flexibility Chart. Strive for optimal flexibility— not too much and not too little.

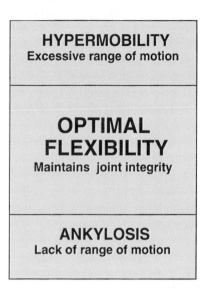

HYPERMOBILITY
Excessive range of motion

OPTIMAL FLEXIBILITY
Maintains joint integrity

ANKYLOSIS
Lack of range of motion

joint in terms of the amount of movement allowed and the direction of movement each joint permits.

The hip and shoulder are ball and socket joints, which possess the greatest range of motion in the body. However, their difference in flexibility is like day and night. The shoulder is the most flexible joint in the body. It is protected primarily by muscle and is considered a loose joint. The shoulder joint is inherently flexible and can be maintained with moderate exercise. In contrast, the hip joint is unable to be as flexible as the shoulder joint. In fact, this would not be desirable because the hip joint must support the weight of the body.

The goal for your stretching program is to maintain joint integrity to stay in the optimal flexibility range (see figure 7.2). Too much or too little is unhealthy. **Hypermobility,** or excessive range of motion, can develop if the connective tissue that surrounds the joint is stretched too far. Hypermobility could lead to a decrease in joint stability and integrity, thereby increasing the susceptibility of that joint to injury. However, no one really knows how much range of motion is too much. On the other hand, a lack of flexibility (**ankylosis**) is also undesirable.

Women tend to be more flexible than men at all ages. Reasons for greater range of motion in women include differences in their skeletal bones, muscle mass, and body composition. Women also do more flexibility exercises than men, giving them an advantage in their range of motion. Some studies have indicated the vulnerability of women to certain injuries because of low joint stability (e.g., dislocation of the kneecap). Most women only require a moderately intense training program to make substantial gains in flexibility.

The safest and most beneficial time to stretch to improve flexibility is right after a workout. This is the time when muscles and joints are warm and can be stretched farther without tearing. The only visible guarantee that deep muscle temperature is sufficiently high for stretching is when you "break a sweat."

Moving a joint only through its full range of motion can be performed safely several times

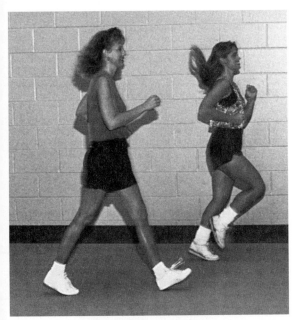

Light muscle activity such as walking and slow jogging can allow for safer and more efficient stretching.

each day. However, pushing the joint beyond its normal range should be performed more carefully and less often. Any stretching done before the deep muscles are warm (like in the warm-up) should be done gently and slowly. Stretching performed later in the day is safer because the joints get warmer from normal movement during the day.

Stretching exercises in the warm-up should be performed after several minutes of light muscle activity. It is highly desirable to warm the muscles up before stretching them. When the muscles contract they generate heat. A warmer muscle temperature allows for safer and more efficient stretching. Slow walking, jogging, or calisthenics are examples of light muscle activity to help raise the muscle temperature.

Weight training can increase flexibility. In a previous Olympics, the U.S. athletes were compared in flexibility. As was expected, the gymnasts were most flexible. The second most flexible group of U.S. Olympic athletes were the weight lifters. To improve flexibility during weight training, the limb being exercised should be moved through a full range of motion. This is for each repetition, and the muscles on both sides of the limb should be equally exercised. Lifting weights correctly will allow a joint to be strengthened and stabilized without significant loss of flexibility.

There are no absolute standards for flexibility. Different movements, activities, and sports require differing amounts of flexibility within a wide variety

of joints. The type of activity you engage in will dictate the amount of flexibility you need to be able to safely participate in that activity.

In the process of aging, flexibility is normally lost. Most adults become less flexible as they grow older. Researchers have not been able to identify, with scientific precision, the reason for this loss of range of motion. They do know that range of motion is lost at a steadily increasing rate as aging continues.

Inactivity is the major cause in the loss of flexibility during the aging process. A fitness program cannot stop aging and its progressively debilitating effects, but it can slow it down. You can maintain at least adequate levels of flexibility throughout your life by an appropriate stretching program.

Permanent loss of flexibility is possible. When a joint is not moved through its full range of motion, the muscles and connective tissue around the joint can shorten, become stiff, and be hard to move. If the shortening (**contracture**), becomes permanent, postural problems may result with accompanying loss of smooth, graceful, fluid movement. The crippling effects of contractures can often be seen in the elderly, but this condition can afflict anyone who has experienced surgery, a cast immobilization, or inactivity for a long time.

METHODS TO DEVELOP FLEXIBILITY

Improving your flexibility requires stretching the muscles crossing the joint and other soft tissues around the joint beyond their normal range. If you only want to maintain your joint's present level of flexibility, you can simply move the joint through its full range of motion.

There are three effective methods for improving flexibility.

1. **Static stretching** is the safest and most preferred way to stretch because it is easy to learn, there is less chance of injury, less energy is required, and it can be performed alone. This is a relaxed, gradual, and sustained stretch. A review of stretching research recommends that individual stretching exercises should be performed **near the end of their range of motion or just to the point where there is a sensation of tightness, but not discomfort.**

   The latest research also recommends **holding the stretch between fifteen and thirty seconds and perform two to four stretches for each muscle group** (see table 7.1 for effective exercise strategies to develop flexibility). An example of static stretching is bending from the waist and slowly

TABLE 7.1

Effective Exercise Guidelines for Developing Flexibility

Type	Static
Frequency	A minimum of 3 times per week
Intensity	Low (a relaxed, gradual, and sustained stretch that you hold at the beginning of tightness). Each stretch should be performed slowly. Over time, strive for a gradual progression to greater ranges of motion.
Time	15 to 30 seconds and 2 to 4 repetitions per muscle group

Note: It is recommended that an active warm-up that includes light activity precede vigorous stretching exercises. If stretching exercises are performed prior to the aerobic workout, they should be used with particular caution.

allowing your hands to reach down as far as your range of motion will allow. When you feel the beginning of tightness, you should hold the stretch there between fifteen and thirty seconds.

2. **Ballistic stretching** consists of bobbing and bouncing movements, such as a series of up-and-down bobs as you attempt to touch your toes. The rapid pace and continuous motion of bobbing and bouncing produces momentum and can stretch the muscle fibers too far. This can lead to injuries in the joint structure.

   Although ballistic stretching is more likely to lead to tears in the joint's soft tissue for the regular exerciser, it can be useful for athletes who are already highly conditioned and used to the vigorous movements. Warming up the muscles first through light activity and static stretching is highly recommended. Then ballistic stretching may be used because it more realistically resembles the reaching and stretching movements performed in athletic competition.

3. **PNF (Proprioceptive Neuromuscular Facilitation)** is a series of contractions and relaxations of a muscle following a maximum contraction of that muscle. It normally requires a partner and more time than the other stretching methods. Also, a maximum isometric contraction can lead to injuries in some people.

   To begin the stretch, your partner moves your particular joint partially through its range of motion. As you begin to feel discomfort from the stretch, you should contract isometrically for a period of four to five seconds against the pressure your partner is applying. After the contraction, briefly relax. Next, allow your partner to move your joint further in its range of motion—stopping again when discomfort is felt.

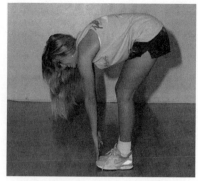

Static stretch

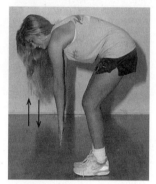

Ballistic stretch

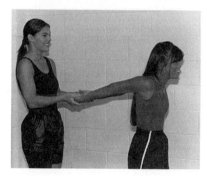

PNF stretch

STRATEGIES TO IMPROVE FLEXIBILITY

Use static stretch (see table 7.1).

Do not injure the soft tissues. You should not experience discomfort or pain while stretching. If you experience any discomfort or pain, you are stretching too far.

Breathe slowly, rhythmically, and comfortably while stretching. Do not hold your breath. If you cannot breathe normally while stretching, you are probably stretching too far.

Stretch any time you feel tightness. Stretching does not have to be restricted only to your workout.

Perform a light activity before you stretch. Be sure your muscles are completely warmed up before performing stretching exercises to increase flexibility.

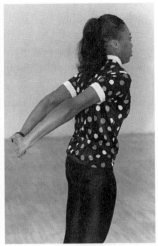

Anterior shoulder stretch

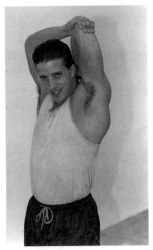

Posterior shoulder stretch

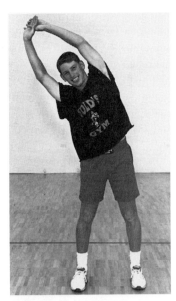

Side stretch

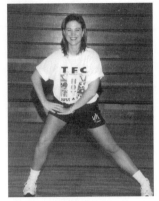

Adductor stretch

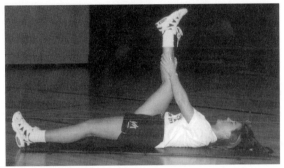

Hamstring stretch

Make stretching a relaxing daily habit. What better way to start your day than to perform a routine of stretches! How about stretching right before you go to bed? It may help you relax and sleep better. And how about before and after your workout? It will improve your performance and reduce your risk for injury.

STRETCHES FOR FLEXIBILITY

1. **Anterior Shoulder Stretch.** Start in a standing position. With your hands behind your back, join the fingers of both hands together. Straighten both arms and raise your hands as high as possible behind your back. Hold this position.

2. **Posterior Shoulder Stretch.** Start in a standing position. Place your right arm overhead with your elbow bent. Grasp your right elbow with your left hand and gently pull your right elbow and upper arm behind your head. Hold this position. Repeat this exercise with the left arm.

3. **Side Stretch.** Stand with your feet shoulder-width apart. Place both arms straight above your head and lean to the left. Stretch all of the muscles along the right side of your body. Hold this position. Repeat this exercise leaning to the right.

4. **Adductor Stretch.** Start in a standing position. Assume a straddle position with your feet apart, approximately two times your shoulder width. Bend your right knee slightly and stretch the muscles along the inside of your left thigh. Hold this position. Repeat this exercise with your left knee slightly bent and stretch the muscles along the inside of your right thigh.

5. **Hamstring Stretch.** Start in a position lying on your back with your knees bent and both feet flat on the floor. Raise your right leg with your knee bent. Grasp behind the calf with both hands. Pull your right leg toward your chest while trying to straighten your leg at the knee. Hold this position. Repeat this exercise using the opposite leg.

6. **Low Back Stretch.** Start in a position lying on your back with both legs straight. Pull one thigh toward your chest with your knee bent and both

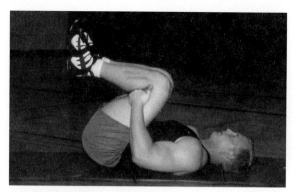

Low back stretch

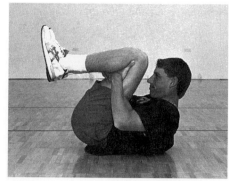

Knees to chest stretch

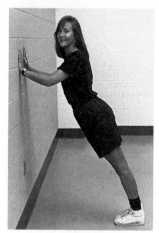

Calf stretch

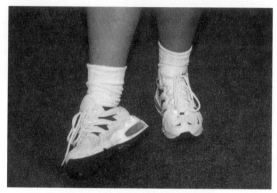

Lateral ankle circle stretch

hands behind your thigh. Hold this position. Repeat this exercise using the opposite leg.

7. **Knees to Chest Stretch.** Start in a position lying on your back with your knees bent and both feet flat on the floor. Bring both knees toward your chest. Grasp the back of both thighs and pull your knees toward your chest while curling your upper body forward. Hold this position.

8. **Calf Stretch.** Stand approximately three feet away from a wall, with your feet about twelve inches apart. Lean forward from the ankles and place your hands on the wall. Keep your body and your legs straight. Lean forward as far as possible while keeping your feet (especially heels) flat on the floor. Hold this position.

9. **Lateral Ankle Circle Stretch.** Stand on your left foot. Rotate your right foot, inverting the ankle. Have the bottom of the foot facing in. Do not invert too far. Hold. Repeat this exercise with the left foot.

MEASURING FLEXIBILITY

No one test will provide an indication of overall body flexibility. Because flexibility measurement must be specific, there are different tests for different joints.

The following section offers four different flexibility tests that are included in Activity 7A. Follow directions carefully for each flexibility test. Table 7.2 provides ratings for the following tests.

Test 1: The Modified Sit-and-Reach Test

This test is designed to measure the flexibility of the lower back and hamstrings. It takes into account differences in arm and leg length.

1. Remove your shoes and sit on the floor with your knees together and your feet (including heels) flat against a bench or sit-and-reach box. The six-inch mark of the measuring stick should be even with the seat of the bench or sit-and-reach box.

2. With your hands one on top of the other, slowly reach forward with your arms fully extended. Reach as far as you can and hold.

3. Have your partner measure the distance your fingertips reach on the measuring stick. Perform the test three times and record the best score.

TABLE 7.2

Ratings for Modified Sit-and-Reach Test, Trunk Extension, Total Body Rotation Test, and Shoulder Lift Flexibility Test

Ratings	Men					Women				
	Sit & Reach	Trunk Extension	Total Body Rotation		Shoulder Lift	Sit & Reach	Trunk Extension	Total Body Rotation		Shoulder Lift
			R	L				R	L	
Good	10+	19+	17+	18+	22+	10+	20+	17+	18+	23+
Fair	6–9	14–18	15–16	15–17	14–21	6–9	14–19	15–16	15–17	15–22
Low	<6	<14	<15	<15	<14	<6	<14	<15	<15	<15

Note: These standards have been designed for the 18- to 26-year-old age group. Younger and older populations may have more difficulty reaching the higher levels of achievement.

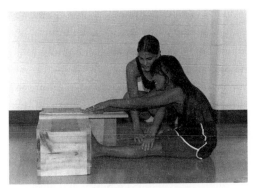

Modified sit-and-reach test

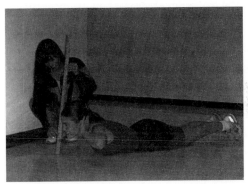

Trunk extension test

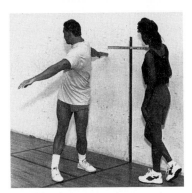

Total body rotation test

Test 2: The Trunk Extension Test

This test is designed to measure your trunk extension.

1. Lie in a prone position on the floor with your hands held behind the head.
2. Hold your hips securely to the floor.
3. Lift the upper body up as far as possible and hold.
4. The recorded score is the number of inches from the chin to the floor.

Test 3: The Total Body Rotation Test

This test is designed to measure trunk rotation.

1. Place a vertical mark or strip of tape on a wall. The vertical line should extend from the floor to a height of seventy-two inches. Place another mark or a strip of tape on the floor. The floor line should be perpendicular to the vertical line and extend thirty-six inches from the wall.
2. Stand at arm's length from the wall with the toes of both feet touching the line on the floor.
3. A partner should hold a measuring stick in a horizontal position against a wall at shoulder height. The fifteen-inch mark of the measuring stick should be even with the vertical line. The zero mark of the measuring stick may be attached to the wall with a strip of tape. However, it will need to be realigned with the shoulder of each subject.
4. Rotate the body so that the shoulder farthest from the wall moves backward. Keep the shoulders in a horizontal plane. Extend the arms and

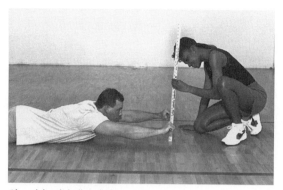

Shoulder lift flexibility test

fingers and move the hand along the measuring stick as far as possible. Be sure to keep the wrist and fingers straight. Repeat from the other side.

5. The highest mark reached on the measuring stick is the score. Measure to the nearest inch. Repeat the test three times and record the best score.

Test 4: The Shoulder Lift Flexibility Test

This test is designed to measure shoulder flexion.

1. Lie down in the prone position on the floor with the arms fully extended forward and parallel.
2. Hold a stick or ruler with both hands. Be sure to keep the elbows and wrists straight.
3. One partner should hold a measuring stick (yardstick) vertically with the zero mark on the floor. Place the measuring stick close enough to get an accurate measurement.
4. Keep the chin on the floor and raise the arms upward as far as possible. Elbows and wrists should be kept straight. For extra stability, have a partner press down gently on the back of the knees.
5. The recorded score is the number of inches from the stick to the floor. Measure to the nearest inch. Repeat the test three times and record the best score.

SUMMARY

- Flexibility, the fourth health-related fitness component, is the amount of movement, or range of motion, you have at each joint. Today, stretching exercises are considered essential to any physical fitness program.

- Being flexible improves your ability to perform daily tasks and makes it possible for you to enjoy a more active lifestyle. On the other hand, limited range of motion of a joint can limit your performance in many activities and will increase the risk of injury to your soft tissue (muscles, tendons, and ligaments).
- Limitations to flexibility are determined by joint structure and the soft tissue around the joint.
- Flexibility is specific to each joint.
- Hypermobility, or range of motion beyond normal, can develop if the connective tissue that surrounds the joint is stretched too far.
- Women tend to be more flexible than men at all ages.
- The safest and most beneficial time to stretch to improve flexibility is right after a workout.
- Moving a joint only through its full range of motion can be performed safely several times each day.
- Stretching is not synonymous with warming up.
- Weight training can increase flexibility.
- There are no absolute standards for flexibility.
- In the process of aging, flexibility is normally lost.
- Inactivity is the major cause in the loss of flexibility during the aging process.
- Permanent loss of flexibility is possible.
- There are three effective methods for improving flexibility.
    1. Static stretching is the safest and most preferred way to stretch. This is a relaxed, gradual, and sustained stretch that should be performed near the end of the range of motion or just to the point where there is a sensation of tightness, but not discomfort. Also, hold the static stretch between fifteen and thirty seconds and perform two to four stretches for each muscle group at least three times a week.
    2. Ballistic stretching consists of bobbing and bouncing movements, such as a series of up-and-down bobs as you attempt to touch your toes.
    3. PNF (Proprioceptive Neuromuscular Facilitation) is a series of contractions and relaxations of a muscle following a maximum contraction of that muscle.
- There are many strategies to follow in a stretching program.
- No one test will provide an indication of overall body flexibility.

ACTIVITY   7A

MEASURING FLEXIBILITY

Name _____   **To be submitted: Yes   No**

Date _____   **If yes, due date** _____

Class _____   Section _____   **Score** _____

PURPOSE
To measure flexibility in the lower back, trunk, and shoulders.

DIRECTIONS
1. Perform the flexibility tests on pages 90 to 92.
2. Record your scores in the Results section.
3. Rate your scores using table 7.2 on page 91 and record the ratings in the Results section.
4. Answer the questions in the Results section.

RESULTS
1. What were your flexibility scores and ratings for the four tests?

	Scores	Ratings
Test 1: Modified Sit-and-Reach Test	_____	_____
Test 2: Trunk Extension Test	_____	_____
Test 3: Total Body Rotation Test	_____	_____
Test 4: Shoulder Lift Flexibility Test	_____	_____

2. How would you evaluate your overall level of flexibility?

3. Do you plan to improve your flexibility?   Yes   No   If yes, what stretches will you use?

A C T I V I T Y   7B

PERFORMING STRETCHING EXERCISES FOR FLEXIBILITY

Name _____   **To be submitted: Yes   No**

Date _____   **If yes, due date _____**

Class _____   Section _____   **Score _____**

PURPOSE
1. To provide some sample stretching exercises that can be used to develop flexibility.
2. To provide you an opportunity to experience a lifetime flexibility program.

DIRECTIONS
1. First, perform an aerobic workout for at least fifteen minutes or until the muscles are warmed.
2. Next, perform all nine flexibility exercises listed on pages 89 to 90.
3. Hold each stretch (except the ankle stretch) for ten seconds at a point of mild discomfort.
4. Follow the guidelines found in table 7.1 on page 88.

RESULTS
1. Did you enjoy performing the nine stretches for developing flexibility?   Yes   No

2. Did you experience any pain while stretching?   Yes   No   If so, where was it located?

3. Do you plan to include a flexibility program as part of your total fitness program?   Yes   No   Explain.

STRATEGIES FOR HEALTHY BODY COMPOSITION

Having the right amount of body fat—not too much and not too little—contributes to health, self-esteem, and a desirable appearance.

LEARNING OBJECTIVES

- Define body composition, percent body fat, and obesity.

- Discuss why overfat is a better indicator of health than overweight.

- Examine the health problems of obesity.

- Describe the five theories of obesity.

- Perform three measurements to assess body composition.

LIFESTYLE QUESTIONS

- Are you satisfied with your present level of body weight?

- Are you satisfied with your present level of body fat?

- Do you know an obese person who has health problems from his or her condition?

INTRODUCTION

Body composition—the fifth component of health-related fitness—refers to the percentage of muscle, fat, bone, and other tissue that the body is made up of. In our society, the two health-related components that most people are concerned about are cardiorespiratory fitness and body composition. Possessing both a fit cardiorespiratory system and a desirable level of body fat can lead to a higher quality of life and less risk for heart disease, cancer, stroke, high blood pressure, and diabetes.

At some time in your life, you have probably been concerned about your body weight and/or body fat. A few of us are happy with it, but most of us want to lose at least a pound or an inch. There are even a few that want to gain weight. **Body esteem,** or the way we feel about our body, is tied to how we feel about our total self. How can we feel better about our body and, in turn, feel better about ourselves? One strategy is to be more active during our day and have a consistent exercise program. Being physically fit will contribute to a healthier body and a more desirable appearance.

In this chapter, body fat—instead of weight—will be the focus. This is because the relationship of excessive body fat to the leading causes of death is well documented. However, being *underfat* has its problems, too. The goal for you in this health-related component of fitness is to maintain a healthy percentage of body fat—not too much and not too little.

OVERWEIGHT

Many people use charts to determine desirable weight. A height and weight chart can provide you with some information about how you compare with population averages. It can also give a general idea about whether you have accumulated too much or too little body weight. For excess weight, medical professionals often use 20 percent above ideal weight as an indicator of obesity. However, this method is not as

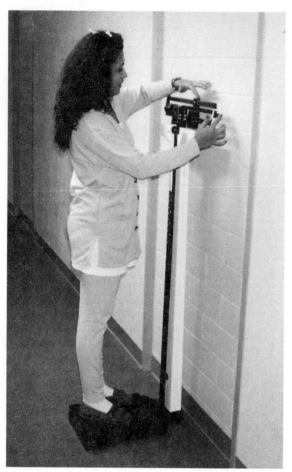

Comparing your weight with population norms is useful to maintain desirable weight but is unreliable as a measurement for good health.

accurate as measuring percent body fat because the extra weight could be composed of muscle tissue.

Although height and weight charts can serve as useful guides to maintaining desirable weight, they are unreliable as measurements for good health. Since height and weight charts represent population averages, they do not provide ideal body weight. As the population has become fatter, the averages on height and weight charts have increased. The adjustments on the charts allows individuals to have more weight and still be considered in the desirable range. Height and weight charts also do not detect levels of percent body fat—a more reliable indicator of good health than pounds on a scale.

PERCENT BODY FAT

The percentage of total body weight that is stored body fat is called percent body fat. The portion of total body weight that is composed of lean tissue,

called **lean body weight,** includes muscles, tendons, bones, and so on. It is a misconception that all body fat is unhealthy, because we each need some stored body fat known as **essential fat.** This level is the minimum amount of body fat needed for good health. Essential fat is required for such important functions as shock absorption for the internal organs, temperature regulation, and transporting the fat-soluble vitamins A, D, E, and K within the body.

Although some fat is essential, an enormous health problem in our society is the number of children, adolescents, and adults who possess too much weight and fat (see table 8.1 for the percent body fat chart).

OBESITY (OVERFATNESS)

Obesity is a condition that indicates the body has stored an excessive amount of body fat. This condition is considered a chronic, degenerative disease that kills people and costs 70 billion dollars annually for fat-related illnesses. There is a lack of accurate data regarding the level at which stored body fat becomes a serious health problem. However, there seems to be general agreement that men with more than 25 percent body fat and women with more than 30 percent body fat should be considered obese.

Besides having high levels of body fat, where people store fat may increase their risk for disease. In fact, where the body fat is located may be even more unhealthy than the amount of excess body fat. An apple-shaped body that stores fat in the abdominal area may be more at risk of heart disease, hypertension, strokes, and diabetes than a pear-shaped body, which stores fat in the hips and thighs.

Creeping obesity is the term used for the gradual process of people accumulating too much body fat for their health. Obesity does not occur overnight; it is months and years in the making. As we age, the extra weight and fat accumulates as we become less active and our basal metabolic rate (BMR) decreases. BMR is the amount of energy expended at rest to sustain the vital functions of the body. For an average person, creeping obesity could result in one-half to one pound of fat gain per year.

UNDERFATNESS

Too little fat can be just as dangerous as too much fat. Females with 8 percent or less and males with 5 percent or less body fat are considered underfat. Although it is important to be aware of the dangers for obesity, excessive concern for thinness can also be a problem. America's obsession for being thin has led

TABLE 8.1
Percent Body Fat Rating Scale

Classification	Men	Women
Essential	no less than 5%	no less than 8%
Desirable % body fat for good performance	6%–13%	9%–22%
Desirable % body fat for good health	14%–25%	23%–30%
Overfat	>25%	>30%

to an increase in eating disorders such as anorexia nervosa, bulimia, and bulimarexia. Each disorder is considered a serious health problem and usually involves the severe restriction of food and/or regurgitation of food. More information on being underfat and eating disorders can be found in chapter 13.

WHY CONTROL WEIGHT AND BODY FAT?

Achieving and maintaining desirable weight and body fat is one important goal of a healthy lifestyle. A healthy body will allow you to live life to the fullest, enjoying family, school, work, and leisure time. However, an obese or too thin body can adversely affect you in all wellness components and lead to a poorer quality of life.

Many physical problems are associated with being obese. Obesity is linked with several heart disease risk factors, including high blood pressure, high cholesterol, and diabetes. Certain cancers, such as breast cancer for women and prostate and colon cancer for men, are prevalent in the obese. Strokes or kidney problems may result from high blood pressure. The obese may also suffer from back pain and degenerative joint diseases like arthritis.

Numerous mental health problems are also linked to being overfat. In America, a social stigma is attached to being obese. The overfat are seen as unattractive, inadequate, unhealthy, undisciplined, insecure, depressed, and having poor personalities. They are also perceived as having higher anxiety levels and having lower self-concepts than normal weight people. These characteristics are certainly not true of everyone who is overfat. Those who find themselves with too much fat, however, are still perceived this way.

Also, as a result of social conditioning, the overfat often encounter teasing, ridicule, and rejection. In turn, psychological problems may result in the form of a poor body image, a sense of failure, a pas-

sive approach to life situations, and an expectation of rejection. Psychologists also think that a person may use fat as a protection from physical and, therefore, emotional relationships with others. Such a person may require therapy to lose weight/fat.

Obesity has also been linked to a shorter life span. Research has indicated that those who are moderately overfat may have a 40 percent higher risk of a shortened life span than those whose body fat levels are healthy. Also, severe obesity may result in a 70 percent higher risk of dying early that those with healthy body fat levels.

THEORIES OF OBESITY

Times are changing. For years, the obese individual was thought to have too little self-control and too much self-indulgence. This idea may partially explain why some become obese, but there is much more to it. New research suggests that the causes of obesity are a combination of genetic, physical, mental, and environmental factors. Several theories have emerged to help explain the challenges of weight and fat control.

The Energy Balance Equation Theory

The energy balance equation theory suggests that calories consumed (energy input) must equal calories expended (energy output) for body weight to remain the same. Any imbalance in calories consumed or calories expended will result in a change in body weight (see figure 8.1). Since one pound of stored body fat is equal to 3,500 calories, you will gain one pound of fat by consuming an extra 3,500 calories. On the other hand, you will also lose one pound of fat by expending an extra 3,500 calories. According to the energy balance theory, the three ways to lose fat are: (1) reduce calories consumed below daily energy requirements, (2) increase your

FIGURE 8.1
The Energy Balance Seesaw

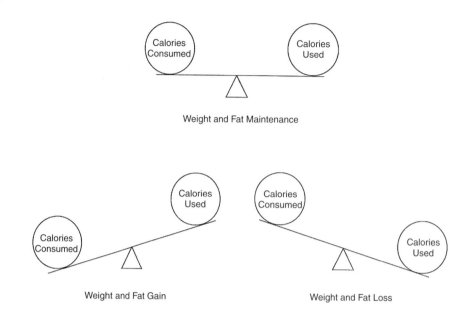

calories expended above energy requirements through physical activity, and, for best results, (3) combine methods 1 and 2.

The Sluggish Metabolism Theory

The sluggish metabolism theory states that the overfat individual, having a lower BMR, requires fewer calories for normal body functions than the normal weight person. Most women require 1,200 to 1,450 calories daily, whereas most men need 1,600 to 1,800 daily calories. Since the overfat appear to have a sluggish BMR, they convert food into energy more slowly, using fewer calories than the normal weight person. Therefore, fewer calories are needed to maintain normal body functions and the unused calories are stored as fat—leading to obesity. Several factors influence your BMR, including genetics, age, gender, body size, nutritional status, body type, and activity level (see figure 8.2).

The Fat Cell Theory

The fat cell theorists believe that the number and size of your fat cells will determine your level of fatness. When the body needs to expand fat storage, it may increase the number and/or size of the fat cells. A normal weight person will have between 25 billion and 30 billion fat cells, whereas an obese person may have four times this number—up to 120 billion. In addition, as fat cells become full, they can expand up to three times their normal size. New fat cells, if needed by the body, can also be formed for energy storage.

FIGURE 8.2
BMR Factors and Their Influence

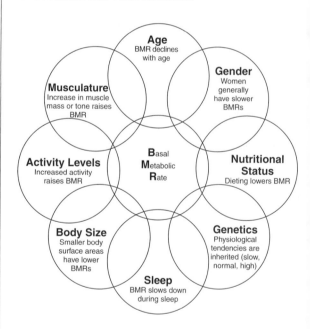

Fat cell development is significantly increased during three critical periods. The three critical periods are during the last trimester of pregnancy, the first year of life, and the adolescent growth spurt. Overfeeding and overeating during the three critical periods may trigger an acceleration of fat cells, increasing the likelihood of adult obesity. New evidence suggests that additional fat cells may be created in adulthood, although not at the same pace as in childhood.

FIGURE 8.3
The Vicious Cycle of Long-Term Dieting and Overeating

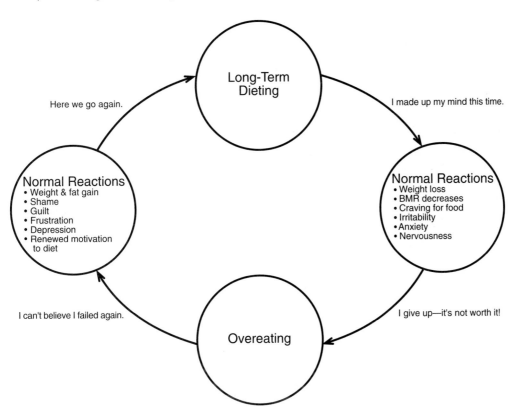

A constant struggle exists between the dieter and the billions of fat cells. A vicious cycle of long-term dieting (weight loss) and overeating (weight gain), called the **yo-yo syndrome,** is set in motion (see figure 8.3). Your body's natural instinct is to maintain the comfort of the fat cells by defending their size. As the fat cells become deprived when dieting, they fight back, causing feelings of irritability, anxiety, and nervousness. The dieter then surrenders to the food cravings caused by the starving fat cells and overeats. Instead of the expected loss, the fat cells become enlarged, resulting in weight and fat gain. This is why more than 90 percent of all dieters eventually gain their weight back within two years. The solution is to shrink the size of the fat cells through increased physical activity.

The Set Point Theory

The set point theory suggests that people have an internal proficiency to control their weight and fat. Why do some people eat like horses without gaining an ounce while others seem to gain pounds by walking past a bakery shop? The answer seems to be linked to your set point. There appears to be a direct link between the amount of stored fat in the body and the body's metabolic rate (the rate at which en-

ergy is used). The body works hard to maintain this stable amount of stored fat. Even after periods of undereating and overeating when weight is lost and gained, the body will adjust its appetite and metabolism rate to return back to its previous weight.

The level of fat storage with which your body is most comfortable is your set point. The hypothalamus gland in your brain regulates the set point by acting as your body's thermostat. Dieting produces a lower amount of fat storage and thereby lowers the set point. When this happens, the hypothalamus switches on, lowering metabolism and producing feelings of hunger. Your body then fights to raise the set point by using calories wisely and crying out to be fed.

Heredity can play a major role with your set point. Through genetics, some individuals will have higher set points, leading to a maintenance of higher body fat levels. Others are given lower set points, leading to a maintenance of lower body fat levels. If your set point is set high and dieting is your only strategy, you may be engaged in an endless battle against your fat cells.

The key is to lower your set point so that your body will be more comfortable with a lower level of fat. The best way to lower your set point and lose unwanted weight and fat is through regular physical exercise and nutritious food selection. When your set point is reduced, your body will increase its metabolism and use more calories at rest. This will make it easier for you to maintain desirable weight and body fat levels.

The Insulin Theory

New studies are showing that the pancreas of the genetically obese appears to oversecrete insulin early in life. Over time, this causes the liver and muscle cells to become insulin-resilient, which only stimulates the body into secreting more insulin. Too much insulin interrupts and slows down the proper metabolism of glucose (our body's energy supply) and inhibits the breakdown and use of body fat for energy. The excess glucose and fat end up being stored in the body's tissues, compounding the problem of losing weight.

STRATEGIES FOR CONTROLLING WEIGHT AND BODY FAT

For a lifetime of weight and fat control, experts now recommend a new lifestyle approach that is more accommodating for the individual. The new plan calls for a flexible, accepting, and family-based program that discourages dieting. The program contains five equal components, each one important to the success of the participant: (1) Get Psyched! (2) Get Nutritionally Aware! (3) Change Unhealthy Behaviors! (4) Get Physically Active! and (5) Get Support! Chapter 13 provides an in-depth discussion of these five strategies to lifetime weight and fat control. See table 8.2 for important exercise strategies to control body fat.

MEASURING BODY FAT

Although body fat cannot be measured with absolute accuracy, several methods of estimating body fat have proven to be fairly reliable and reasonably accurate. Methods for estimating percent body fat include underwater weighing, water displacement, X ray, ultrasound, electrical impedance, body girth, and skinfold measurement. Of these, skinfold measurement is one of the least expensive, most accurate, and most available methods.

About 50 percent of body fat is stored just beneath the skin. The other 50 percent is distributed around the various organs and in the muscles. Skinfold calipers are used to measure the thickness of a fold of skin and the fat located directly under it. Taken at different body sites, the thickness of the skinfolds can be used to obtain a good estimate of total body fatness (see Activity 8A).

Body girth measurements are less reliable than skinfold measurements but are easy to perform. Like height and weight charts, girth measurements should be used with caution. If used as a secondary source of reference, this measurement can be beneficial.

ASSESSING YOUR BODY FATNESS, CIRCUMFERENCE, AND WEIGHT

Guidelines for Skinfold Measurements

1. All skinfold measurements should be made on the right side of the body.
2. The skinfold should be picked up between the thumb and index finger.
3. Measure the thickness of the skinfold approximately one centimeter from the fingers and at a depth that is equal to the thickness of the fold.
4. Make three measurements at each skinfold site. Use the average of the three measurements as the skinfold thickness for that site.
5. Release and regrasp the skinfold for each measurement.

TABLE 8.2
Strategies for Controlling Body Fat

	Lower Limit	Upper Limit
Frequency:	5 days	7 days
Intensity:	60% of working heart rate	80% of working heart rate
Time:	30 min.	60 min.
Type:	Aerobic with strength training	Aerobic/Anaerobic with strength training

Note: Walking is an excellent aerobic activity for controlling body fat because it is low-impact, convenient, and enjoyable.

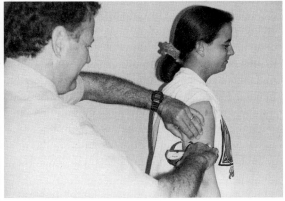
Triceps skinfold

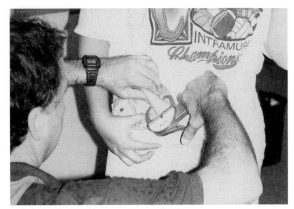
Iliac crest skinfold

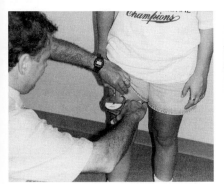
Thigh skinfold

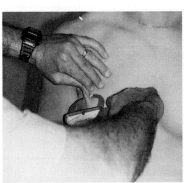
Chest skinfold

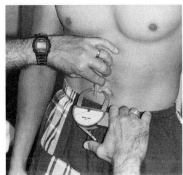
Abdomen skinfold

6. Measurements made by two different people may vary slightly. If you are measured a second time, have the measurements made by the same person at the same time of day.

Skinfold Sites

To determine percent body fat for women, use the sum of the skinfold measurements at the triceps, iliac crest, and thigh. To determine percent body fat for men, use the sum of the skinfold measurements at the chest, abdomen, and thigh.

Triceps Skinfold: Locate a point on the back of the upper arm that is halfway between the top of the shoulder and the tip of the elbow. Measure a vertical skinfold.

Iliac Crest: Locate a point on the side of the waist above the crest of the hip bone and slightly toward the front of the body where there is a natural diagonal skinfold.

Thigh: Locate a point on the front of the thigh halfway between the hip joint and the knee joint. Measure a vertical skinfold.

Chest: Locate a diagonal fold halfway between the front of the armpit and the nipple (for men).

Abdomen: Locate a point that is one inch to the right of the umbilicus and measure a vertical skinfold.

Use of the Nomogram

Add up your three skinfold measurements and mark this sum of skinfolds on the appropriate line of the **nomogram** (a special chart that can be used to determine percent body fat). Place a mark at your age on the nomogram (see fig. 8.4). Use a straight edge to connect these two points. Mark the place where the straight edge crosses the correct percent body fat line for your sex. What is your percent body fat?

Hip-to-Waist Circumference Ratios

Follow these steps in making measurements and calculating hip-to-waist ratios.

1. General guidelines: Use a nonelastic measuring tape. The measurements should be taken with both feet together in the standing position. The arms will be at the sides and raised only enough to allow the measurements. The tape should be horizontal around the entire circumference and pulled snugly but without any indentation. For both measurements, record scores to the nearest millimeter or 1/16 of an inch.
2. Hip Measurement: Measure at the maximum circumference of the buttocks or where you are the largest in the hip area. Wearing bulky clothing may add to the measurement.

FIGURE 8.4

Nomogram to Estimate Percent Body Fat

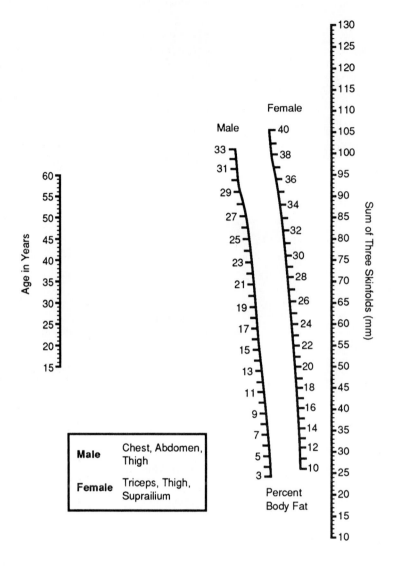

3. Waist Measurement: Measure at the natural waist. If the participant has no natural waist, measure at the level of the umbilicus. Measurement should be made at the end of a normal inhalation.
4. Divide the hip measurement into the waist measurement to determine your ratio.
5. Use table 8.3 to determine your rating for the hip-to-waist ratio.

Height and Weight Measurements

1. Measure your height in inches without wearing shoes and socks.
2. Measure your weight. The chart in table 8.4 is based on weight without clothing. If clothing and/or shoes are worn during the measurement, subtract this weight (1–3 pounds).

3. The higher weights in the ranges generally apply to men, who tend to have more muscle and bone; the lower weights more often apply to women, who have less muscle and bone.

SUMMARY

- Obesity creates many physical, psychological, and financial problems in the United States.
- Body composition refers to the fat and nonfat components of the body.
- Percent body fat is the percentage of total body weight that is composed of fat tissue and is a better indicator for health than body weight.

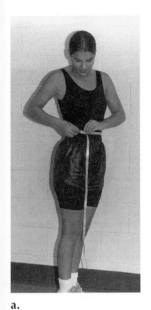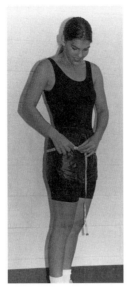

a.   b.

Circumference measurements: (a) Waist (b) Hip

TABLE 8.3

Hip-to-Waist Ratio Rating Scale

Classification	Men	Women	Recommendation
High risk	>1.0	>.85	*Lose weight and fat*
Moderately high risk	.90–1.0	.80–.85	*Lose weight and fat*
Lower risk	<.90	<.80	*None*

Source: Data from Van Itallie, 1988.

TABLE 8.4

Recommended Body Weight Chart

Height	19–34 Years	35 Years and Over	Height	19–34 Years	35 Years and Over
5'0"	97–128	108–138	5'10"	132–174	146–188
5'1"	101–132	111–143	5'11"	136–179	151–194
5'2"	104–137	115–148	6'0"	140–184	155–199
5'3"	107–141	119–152	6'1"	144–189	159–205
5'4"	111–146	122–157	6'2"	148–195	164–210
5'5"	114–150	126–162	6'3"	152–200	168–216
5'6"	118–155	130–167	6'4"	156–205	173–222
5'7"	121–160	134–172	6'5"	160–211	177–228
5'8"	125–164	138–178	6'6"	164–216	182–234
5'9"	129–169	142–183			

The higher weights generally apply to men who tend to have more muscle and bone; the lower weights more often apply to women.

SOURCE: Dietary Guidelines for Americans. Washington, DC: U.S. Department of Agriculture and Department of Health and Human Services, 1990.

- Lean body weight is the portion of total body weight that is composed of lean tissue, which includes muscles, tendons, bones, and so on.
- Body fat is the culprit linked to numerous physical and psychological problems.
- Societal pressure to be thin has led to eating disorders such as anorexia, bulimia, and bulimarexia.
- New research suggests that the causes of obesity are a combination of genetic, physical, mental, and environmental factors.

- Several theories have emerged to help explain the challenges of weight and fat management: energy balance equation, sluggish metabolism, fat cell, set point, and insulin.
- Strategies for lifetime weight and fat control are (1) Get Psyched! (2) Get Nutritionally Aware! (3) Change Unhealthy Behaviors! (4) Get Physically Active! and (5) Get Support!
- Many techniques can be used to measure body fat. A common, reliable method is the use of skinfold measurements.

ACTIVITY 8

DETERMINING BODY FAT, HIP-TO-WAIST RATIO, AND HEALTHY WEIGHT

Name _____   To be submitted: Yes   No

Date _____   If yes, due date _____

Class _____   Section _____   Score _____

PURPOSE

1. To estimate your percent body fat using skinfold measurements.

2. To evaluate your hip-to-waist ratio using circumference measurements.

3. To determine if your weight falls into the recommended weight range.

DIRECTIONS

1. Determine your percent body fat by reading the guidelines for making skinfold measurements described on pages 102 and 103.

2. Determine your hip-to-waist ratio by reading the guidelines on pages 103 and 104.

3. Evaluate your body weight by referring to the recommended weight chart found on page 105.

4. Refer to figure 8.4 on page 104 to determine your percent body fat and table 8.1 on page 99 to determine your rating. Refer to table 8.3 on page 105 to determine your hip-to-waist ratio rating.

5. Record measurements and ratings in the Results section.

6. Answer the questions in the Results section.

RESULTS

1. Write your measurements in the spaces provided. If time is limited, all measurements may not be possible.

Skinfolds (Males)	Partner	Instructor		*Skinfolds (Females)*	Partner	Instructor
Chest	_____	_____		Tricep	_____	_____
Abdominal	_____	_____		Iliac Crest	_____	_____
Thigh	_____	_____		Thigh	_____	_____
Sum	_____	_____		Sum	_____	_____
Percent Body Fat	_____			Percent Body Fat	_____	
Ratings	_____			Ratings	_____	

Circumferences (Males)

Hip Circumference _____

Waist Circumference _____

Hip-to-Waist Ratio _____

Rating _____

Circumferences (Females)

Hip Circumference _____

Waist Circumference _____

Hip-to-Waist Ratio _____

Rating _____

Height and Weight (Males)

Height _____

Weight _____

Within Range?   Yes   No

Height and Weight (Females)

Height _____

Weight _____

Within Range?   Yes   No

(See table 8.4)

1. Were you surprised with your percent body fat level?   Yes   No   Explain.

2. Is your hip-to-waist ratio favorable for lowering risk of disease?   Yes   No   Explain.

3. Is your weight within the healthy ranges recommended for adults?   Yes   No

9

STRATEGIES TO EXERCISE SAFELY

Be a safe exerciser—take the proper precautions!

LEARNING OBJECTIVES

- Explore the dangers and preventive measures for exercising in extreme weather conditions.

- Examine the importance of exercise to back care.

- Discuss strategies to prevent exercise-related injuries.

- Explain the R.I.C.E. formula for the initial treatment of minor injuries.

- Identify the exercises that have been found to be unsafe.

LIFESTYLE QUESTIONS

- Have you ever exercised in extreme hot or cold temperatures? If yes, what measures did you take to be safe?

- Have you ever had back trouble? If yes, what was the cause? And how did you overcome it?

- Do you know an older adult who exercises regularly? If yes, does this individual appear younger than his or her biological years?

- Have you ever had an exercise-related injury? If yes, which one(s)?

- Have you ever performed any of the unsafe exercises found in the last section of this chapter?

INTRODUCTION

Exercise has been touted as a behavior that contributes to numerous fitness and health benefits. However, to ensure these benefits and to be a safe exerciser, there are special considerations in a physical fitness program that deserve attention. Careful thought should be given to exercising in extreme temperature conditions, care of the back, exercising as an older adult, prevention and treatment of injuries, and unsafe exercises (see fig. 9.1).

EXERCISE AND THE ENVIRONMENT

Exercising in extreme weather conditions can lead to serious health problems. Extreme weather conditions such as hot and cold temperatures, humid condi-

tions, and wet weather are legitimate dangers for exercisers. However, if you know the dangers and take precautions, the environment should rarely be an excuse for not exercising.

Hot Weather

The dangers of exercising in hot weather should be taken seriously. During exercise, a loss of body fluid can impair performance. Those who are poorly conditioned, overfat, older, and not acclimatized to exercise in the heat have a higher risk for health problems. People who have previously suffered from heat disorders should be especially careful. Since body temperature must be maintained within a normal range, people who exercise in the heat are most vulnerable to heat stress. Heat-related problems have the greatest chance of occurring when the sun is out and the temperature and relative humidity are high. (See

FIGURE 9.1
Special Considerations for Being a Safe Exerciser

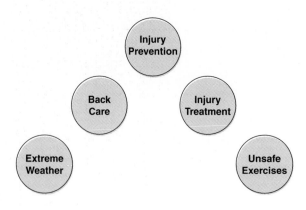

table 9.1) However, they can also occur anytime the body's ability to dissipate heat is impaired.

Hot and humid weather can hamper the body's natural cooling system. To maintain normal body temperature, your body releases heat through sweating and becomes cooled when that sweat evaporates. During exercise, or even when outdoors in hot conditions, your body will tend to perspire or sweat. Sweat won't evaporate well in high humidity, and the coating on the skin can actually cause the body to retain heat.

If your body sweats excessively or there is a lack of fluid replacement such as drinking water, dehydration can result. A dehydrated person stops sweating so evaporation is no longer effective in cooling the body. The body will respond to this heat stress by diverting the blood to the blood vessels in

TABLE 9.1
Exercise in the Heat (Apparent Temperatures)

(To read the table, find the air temperature on the bottom, then find the humidity on the left. Find the apparent temperature where the columns meet.)

□ = Safe Zone
▨ = Caution Zone
▧ = Danger Zone

"Apparent Temperatures"

Relative Humidity (%)	70	75	80	85	90	95	100	105	110	115	120
100	72	80	91	108	132						
95	71	79	89	105	128						
90	71	79	88	102	122						
85	71	78	87	99	117	141					
80	71	78	86	97	113	136					
75	70	77	86	95	109	130					
70	70	77	85	93	106	124	144				
65	70	76	83	91	102	119	138				
60	70	76	82	90	100	114	132	149			
55	69	75	81	89	98	110	126	142			
50	69	75	81	88	96	107	120	135	150		
45	68	74	80	87	95	104	115	129	143		
40	68	74	79	86	93	101	110	123	137	151	
35	67	73	79	85	91	98	107	118	130	143	
30	67	73	78	84	90	96	104	113	123	135	148
25	66	72	77	83	88	94	101	109	117	127	139
20	66	72	77	82	87	93	99	105	112	120	130
15	65	71	76	81	86	91	97	102	108	115	123
10	65	70	75	80	85	90	95	100	105	111	116
5	64	69	74	79	84	88	93	97	102	107	111
0	64	69	73	78	83	87	91	95	99	103	107

Air Temperature (Degrees F)

Source: Data from the National Oceanic and Atmospheric Administration.

TABLE 9.2
Strategies to Prevent Heat-Related Disorders

1. **To stay hydrated and prevent being thirsty, drink plenty of water before, during, and after exercise.** Begin to drink water about thirty minutes before exercising. Continue to drink water frequently during your workout. After exercising, drink as much water as you want. Especially during exercise, you should not allow yourself to feel thirsty. Feeling thirsty is a sign that your body has already lost 2% of its fluids. Although many sports drinks are on the market, plain water is hard to beat as a replacement fluid. Besides being absorbed quickly, it is generally the most available and least expensive. For exercising lasting longer than one or two hours, sport drinks can be beneficial.

2. **Acclimate yourself!** Acclimatization or gradually letting yourself get used to hot and humid environments takes about five to seven days of increasing exposure to heat during exercise. Being in good physical shape and drinking plenty of fluids can accelerate this process.

3. **Properly dress for exercise in hot weather.** Wearing light-colored, lightweight, and loose-fitting clothing will help reflect the sun's rays and allow air to circulate next to your skin. Use a porous hat to allow heat to escape from your head.

4. **Always use your good judgment during hot weather!** Choose a time that is not within the hottest parts of the day, usually from 11:00 A.M. to 4:00 P.M. If you workout outdoors, you can choose to decrease both your intensity and amount of time you exercise. Also, you can plan to rest at regular intervals, preferably in the shade. Or you can exercise indoors. Whether outside or inside, watch for signs of heat stress. If they appear, stop immediately and seek relief.

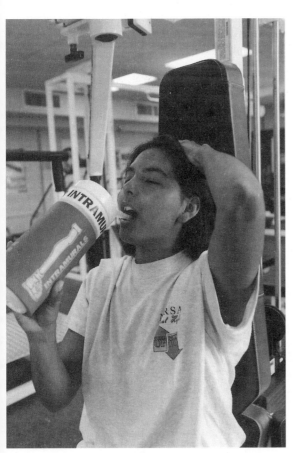

Drink plenty of water before, during, and after exercise.

an attempt to cool the body by exchanging heat directly with the outside environment. This can lead to heat exhaustion, the most severe of all heat-related disorders. Table 9.2 highlights strategies to prevent your risk of heat-related disorders. Figure 9.2 examines the symptoms and treatment strategies for the heat-related disorders of heat cramps, heat exhaustion, and heat stroke.

Cold Weather

The dangers of exercising in cold weather should be taken seriously. Besides being a problem in hot weather, dehydration is also a danger when exercising in cold weather. Your body loses fluids more quickly than you realize. Perspiration is quickly evaporated when the weather is cold and dry. Frostbite is another danger that is associated with cold weather. It can occur within minutes on your hands, nose, ears, and toes but can be avoided with the proper precautions. In cold weather, the windchill factor—the combination of cold temperatures and windy conditions—presents the greatest danger for exercisers (see table 9.3).

You can use many strategies to be a safe exerciser in cold temperatures (see table 9.4).

Wet Weather

Exercising during wet weather can add variety to your fitness program. Rain can be invigorating and exercising in it is a nice break from exercising in dry weather. Exercising in thunderstorms, however, is an entirely different matter. If there is lightning, find a

FIGURE 9.2

Symptoms and Treatments for Heat-Related Disorders

HEAT CRAMPS

SYMPTOMS
Muscle cramps in muscles used most in exercise

TREATMENT
Drink plenty of water, mild stretching, ice massage

HEAT EXHAUSTION

SYMPTOMS
Fatigue, muscle cramps, nausea, headaches, clammy skin, dizziness, paleness, rapid breathing

TREATMENT
Stop exercise, rest in cool place, take off unneeded clothing, drink plenty of water, use cold towels to lower body temp

HEAT STROKE

SYMPTOMS
Fatigue, hot and dry skin, lack of sweating, confusion, fast pulse, high body temperatures, possible seizures, unconsciousness

TREATMENT
Seek immediate medical help. Use every first-aid strategy to immediately lower body temperature

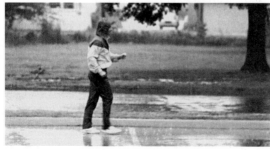

Exercising in the rain can add variety to your exercise program.

way to exercise indoors for that day or at least until the bad weather passes. If you wish to stay dry while exercising in the rain, waterproof exercise suits are available. Although the costs for some are expensive, the water-resistant suits are worth it if they will promote adherence to your exercise program.

CARE OF THE BACK

Careful attention to the back is important in preventing backaches while engaging in an exercise program. Eighty percent of Americans will receive care from a physician for their backs. You may have already experienced back pain in your life. If not, there is a good chance you will. The backache has been called the twentieth-century epidemic, because it is second only to the headache as a common medical complaint. Back problems are the most common cause of inactivity in people under age forty-five.

There are several common causes of backaches. Backaches can be triggered by incorrect postures when studying, working, lying, standing, and sitting. Improper exercises such as straight-knee toe touches and arching the back during bench presses are other factors. In addition, tight back and weak abdominal muscles combined with short hamstring and hip flexor muscles are culprits in back pain.

Physical activity is one of the most common prescriptions for prevention of back pain. Prevention of back problems begins with a physical fitness program that includes aerobic exercise. A program for back care should include flexibility exercises that are important for developing long hamstring and hip flexor muscles (see the following back care exercises). Muscle strength and muscle endurance exercises are also important for a healthy back because they strengthen back and abdominal muscles.

Exercise is often used in recovery for back pain. It can help correct some of the underlying causes by strengthening weak muscles and stretching short ones. Restoring muscle balance relieves muscle spasms by improving postural alignment and body mechanics.

Exercises for a Healthy Back
1. **Arm Lift**
   Starting Position: Lie prone with your forehead resting on the floor and your arms in a reverse T position.
   Movement: Maintaining arm position, lift the arms as high as possible without raising your head or upper body. Hold for ten seconds. Relax and repeat.

TABLE 9.3
Wind-Chill Factor Chart

Estimated Wind Speed (mph)	Actual Thermometer Reading (°F)											
	50	40	30	20	10	0	–10	–20	–30	–40	–50	–60
	Equivalent Temperature (°F)											
Calm	50	40	30	20	10	0	–10	–20	–30	–40	–50	–60
5	48	37	27	16	6	–5	–15	–26	–36	–47	–57	–68
10	40	28	16	4	–9	–24	–33	–46	–58	–70	–83	–95
15	36	22	9	–5	–18	–32	–45	–58	–72	–85	–99	–112
20	32	18	4	–10	–25	–39	–53	–67	–82	–96	–110	–124
25	30	16	0	–15	–29	–44	–59	–74	–88	–104	–118	–133
30	28	13	–2	–18	–33	–48	–63	–79	–94	–109	–125	–140
35	27	11	–4	–20	–35	–51	–67	–82	–98	–113	–129	–145
40	26	10	–6	–21	–37	–53	–69	–85	–100	–116	–132	–148
	Green				Yellow			Red				
(Wind speeds greater than 40 mph have little additional effect.)	LITTLE DANGER (for properly clothed person). Maximum danger of false sense of security.				INCREASING DANGER Danger from freezing of exposed flesh.			GREAT DANGER				

Adapted from Runner's World, 8 (1973):28.

TABLE 9.4
Strategies for Exercising Safely in Cold Temperatures

1. **Drink plenty of water.** Even though you may not feel thirsty, drink liquids before, during, and after exercise. It is also a good idea to avoid diuretic liquids such as coffee and tea before exercise because they can cause frequent urination.

2. **Wear layers of clothing.** Wear light clothing in several layers instead of one heavy garment. With layers, you can peel a layer off if you get too hot. The layer of clothing next to your skin should be absorbent, like a long sleeve T-shirt. A porous windbreaker will help prevent the wind from cooling your body and will allow your body heat to be released.

3. **To prevent frostbite, cover your hands, ears, nose, and feet, because these areas are the most vulnerable.** Use a woolen hat or mask and mittens instead of gloves, since they work the best. If you notice any tissue that is numb or turning hard and white, take immediate action. Get indoors where the air temperature is warmer and soak the tissue in warm water. Avoid hot water because tissue damage may occur.

4. **Avoid getting wet.** Getting wet will cause your body to become colder.

5. **Stay indoors.** Instead of braving the elements, you can choose to exercise in a fitness center or indoor mall. You can also use exercise equipment in your room, apartment, or home.

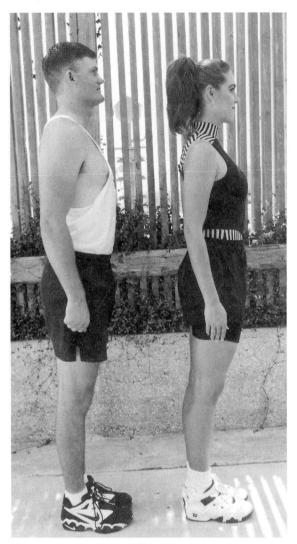

Correct posture for standing

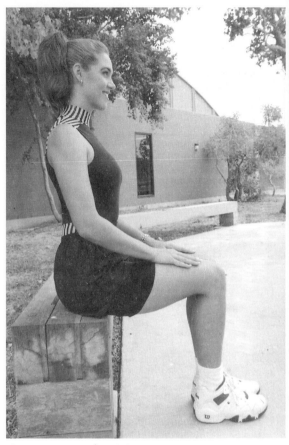

Correct posture for sitting

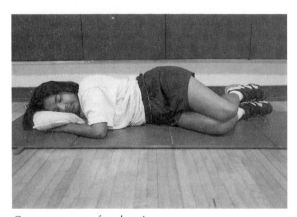

Correct posture for sleeping

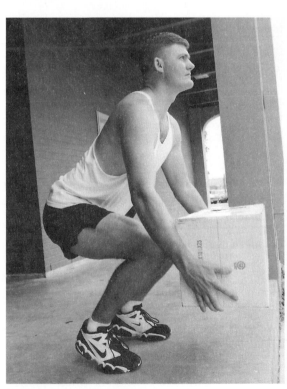

Correct posture for lifting

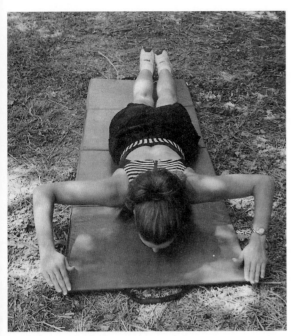

Arm lift

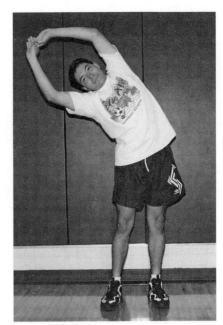

Side stretch

2. **Side Stretch**
   Starting Position: Stand with your feet shoulder-width apart. Place both arms straight above your head.
   Movement: Lean to the left and stretch all of the muscles along the right side of your body. Hold for ten seconds. Switch sides and lean to the right. Repeat.

3. **Hamstring Stretch**
   Starting Position: Lie on your back with your knees bent and both feet flat on the floor.
   Movement: Raise your right leg with your knee bent. Grasp the front of the right foot with your right hand. Place your left hand behind your right knee. Pull your right thigh toward your chest while trying to straighten your leg at the knee. Hold this position for ten seconds. Switch legs. Repeat.

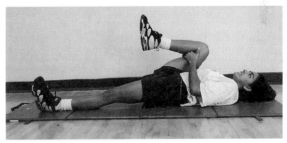

Hamstring stretch

4. **Low Back Stretch**
   Starting Position: Lie on your back with both legs straight.
   Movement: Pull one thigh toward your chest with your knee bent and both hands behind your thigh. Hold for ten seconds. Switch legs. Repeat.

5. **Trunk Curl with Twist**
   Starting Position: Lie supine with your knees bent at 90-degree angles.
   Movement: Flatten lower back and curl head, neck, and shoulders until shoulder blades leave the floor. Twist upper trunk and lift left shoulder higher than right. Reach past right knee with left arm. Hold. Return and repeat with the opposite side.

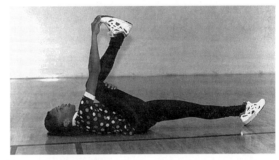

Low back stretch

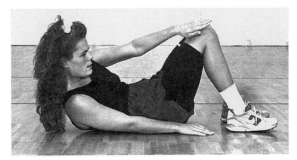

Trunk curl with twist

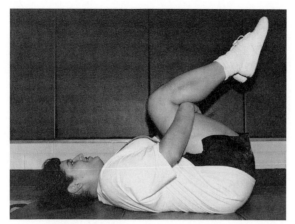

Knees to chest stretch

6. **Knees to Chest Stretch**
   Starting Position: Lie on your back with your knees bent and both feet flat on the floor.
   Movement: Bring both knees toward your chest. Grasp the back of both thighs and pull your knees toward your chest while curling your upper body forward. Hold for ten seconds. Repeat.

7. **Trunk Twist**
   Starting Position: Stand straight, place your feet together, and extend your arms straight out from your sides.
   Movement: Rotate your body as far as possible to one side, keeping your feet stationary. Hold for ten seconds, then rotate your body to the opposite side. Repeat.

8. **Pelvic Tilt**
   Starting position: Supine with knees bent.
   Movement: Tighten the abdominal muscles and tilt the pelvis backward and try to flatten the lower back against the floor. At the same time, tighten the hip and thigh muscles. Hold, then relax. Breathe normally throughout the exercise.

9. **Bridging**
   Starting Position: Supine with knees bent and feet close to buttocks.
   Movement: Contract gluteals, lifting buttocks and lower back off the floor. Hold, then relax, and repeat. Your lower back should not arch.

10. **Sitting Tucks**
    Starting Position: Sit down with your back and feet off the floor and your legs uncrossed.
    Movement: Keeping your feet and back off the floor, alternately draw your legs to your chest and extend them away from your body. Start off with a low number and progress over time.

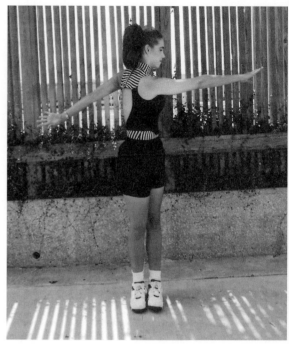

Trunk twist

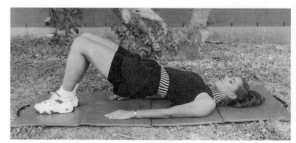

Bridging

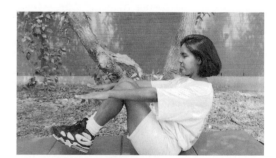

Sitting tucks: starting position

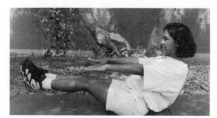

Sitting tucks: extending legs

PREVENTING INJURIES

Although participating in fitness activities can offer many wellness benefits, it can also increase your risk of injury. It is important to note, however, that the benefits far outweigh the risks. When exercising, you intentionally stress certain muscles to increase their strength and stamina. As your body adapts to the new workload, you may experience muscle aches and pains that will usually go away in a short time. Exercise also carries some risk of injury. Chances are, if you are a regular exerciser, over time you will receive a minor or major injury or both. Fortunately, most of these injuries are minor discomforts, and you can resume your workout within a short time. Although no one enjoys being injured or the pain and time off that accompany an injury, the benefits of exercise are so strong that exercisers usually can't wait to get back to their fitness program. (Table 9.5 highlights the four main reasons why injuries occur.)

Prevention is the key to avoid or at least minimize the incidence of injuries. To prevent yourself from being injured, see table 9.6.

TABLE 9.5
Main Causes of Injuries

1. **Overuse**—Injuries can result from exercising too much too soon or exercising too often.

2. **Weakness and inflexibility**—Muscles are either so weak or so tight that unusual twists can strain them.

3. **Mechanical problems**—Caused by improper technique. For example, the way the foot hits the ground while jogging or using too much arm and not enough body in racquet sports.

4. **Footwear**—Wearing incorrect or worn-out shoes.

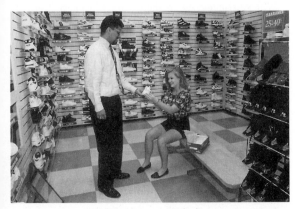

Wearing the proper footwear can help prevent injuries.

INITIAL TREATMENT OF INJURIES

Regardless of which type of injury exercisers encounter, swelling will be a common symptom. Common injuries where swelling occurs range from sprains and strains to tendinitis, bursitis, and muscle soreness. Swelling is most likely to occur during the first seventy-two hours after an injury. The healing process is significantly slowed when swelling occurs, and the injured area will not be able to return to normal until the swelling is gone. Consequently, first-aid management for any acute injury is directed toward controlling the swelling. Rehabilitation time will be significantly reduced if the swelling can be controlled immediately.

TABLE 9.6
Strategies for Injury Prevention

1. Unless you're a trained athlete under supervision, follow the strategies for effective exercising in chapter 4.

2. Always warm up before and cool down after engaging in any fitness program.

3. Set realistic fitness goals.

4. When beginning a physical fitness program, start at a low intensity and gradually progress within your own individual limits. Avoid exercising too much too soon or too often.

5. A good formula for progression is to increase the time of your workout to no more than 10 percent weekly.

6. Cross-train. Cross-training is the use of more than one aerobic activity to achieve cardiorespiratory endurance. Runners can use swimming, cycling, or rowing to periodically replace running in their workout program. Cross-training offers a refreshing change of pace while allowing certain muscles to rest and injuries to heal.

7. Listen to your body during and after exercise. If you develop excessive soreness or pain from exercise, stop immediately. Then for your next workout, choose to either cut back, use a different activity, or even take some time off. If the pain persists, see a physician.

8. Select the appropriate clothing and drink plenty of fluids for exercising in hot, humid, or cold environments.

9. Select and use only high-quality, reliable exercise equipment.

10. Always use your good sense! Avoid improper exercises and exercising alone at night. Also, be cautious exercising around cars, bicycles, dogs, and uneven surfaces.

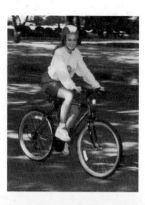

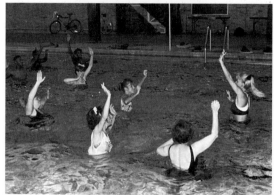

To add variety and prevent injuries, use cross-training activities such as bicycling and swimming in your normal exercise program.

The R.I.C.E. formula is recommended for reducing the initial inflammation and alleviating pain. All four principles should be applied simultaneously.

Rest—You should rest the injured body part for at least seventy-two hours before beginning a rehabilitation program.

Ice—Apply ice to the injured area for fifteen to twenty minutes and repeat every few hours until the swelling disappears. Let the injured area return to a normal temperature between icings and do not apply ice to an area for more than twenty minutes. Apply the ice in a plastic bag.

Compression—Wrap the injured area firmly with an elastic wrap. If the area starts throbbing or begins to change color, the bandage may be wrapped too tightly. It is not recommended to sleep with the wrap on.

Elevation—Lift the injured area above heart level to decrease the blood supply and reduce swelling.

Note: A detailed discussion of injuries encountered by exercisers is beyond the scope of this text. However, if you desire information on exercise-related injuries and their rehabilitation, contact an athletic trainer, physical therapist, or a physician.

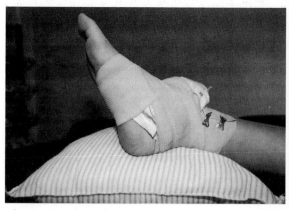

The R.I.C.E. formula: rest, ice, compression, and elevation.

UNSAFE EXERCISES

Many types of exercise place excessive stresses, strains, or compression forces on particular muscles or joints. Unsafe exercises can increase the likelihood for injury to these sites and should be avoided in a physical fitness program. *The following popular exercises have been found to be unsafe and should be avoided.*

1. **Straight-leg lifts** are used to strengthen abdominal muscles and hip flexors. Unsafe because they can put excessive stress on the spine.
2. **Back hyperextensions** are used to strengthen lower back muscles and stretch abdominal muscles. Unsafe because they can place excessive strain on the spine.
3. **Donkey kicks** are used to develop the extensor muscles of the lower back. Unsafe because they place excessive strain on the spine.
4. **Bench presses** are used to improve strength in the pectoral and triceps muscles. Unsafe with feet on the floor and back arched because they place excessive strain on the back.
5. **Sit-ups** are used to strengthen abdominal muscles. Unsafe when hands are placed behind the neck, because they can hyperflex the head and neck, stretching the cervical spine.
6. **Straight-leg sit-ups** strengthen the abdominal muscles. Unsafe because they can cause a forward tilt of the pelvis, placing too much strain on the lower back.
7. **Shoulder-stand bicycling** is used to strengthen the abdominal muscles. Unsafe because it places excessive strain on the neck and upper back.
8. **Standing toe-touches** are used to stretch the hamstring muscles. Unsafe because they can cause the knees to hyperextend and place too much pressure on the lower back.

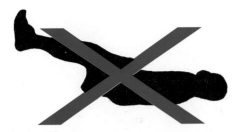

Straight-leg lifts

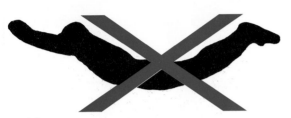

Back hyperextensions

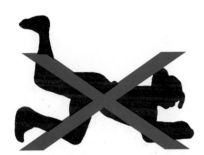

Donkey kicks

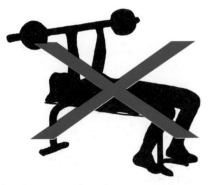

Example of incorrect bench press

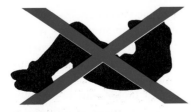

Example of an incorrect sit-up

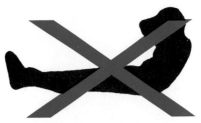

Example of a straight-leg sit-up

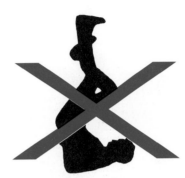

Shoulder-stand bicycling

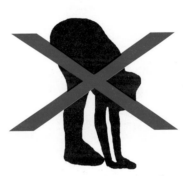

Standing toe-touches

9. **Deep knee bends** are used to strengthen hip and knee extensors. Unsafe because they place extreme stress on the knee area.
10. **Bar stretch** is used to stretch hamstring muscles. Unsafe because it places excessive strain on the knee and can irritate the sciatic nerve.
11. **Hurdler's stretch** is used to stretch the quadriceps muscle. Unsafe because it can cause stress to the ligaments and cartilage within the knee.
12. **Neck circles** are used to develop flexibility in the neck. Unsafe because they cause excessive strain in the disks within the neck.
13. **Quadriceps stretch** is used to stretch the quadriceps muscle. When the knee is hyperflexed 120 degrees or more, it can place excessive strain on the knee, possibly causing cartilage damage.
14. **Knee pull-down** is intended to stretch the lower back. Placing the arms or hands on top of the shin to pull the leg into the body can place undue stress on the knee joint.

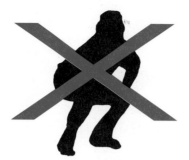

Deep knee bends

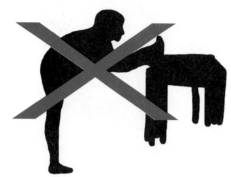

Bar stretch

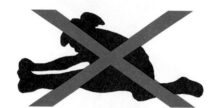

Hurdler's stretch

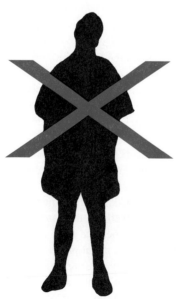

Neck circles

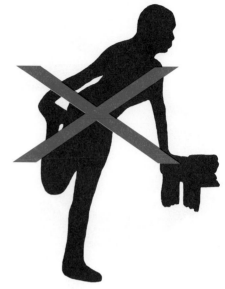

Quadriceps stretch

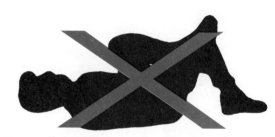

Knee pull-down

SUMMARY

- Extreme weather conditions such as hot and cold temperatures, humid conditions, and wet weather are legitimate dangers for exercisers.
- The environment should rarely be an excuse for not exercising if you know the dangers and take precautions.
- Hot and humid weather can hamper the body's natural cooling system. If your body sweats excessively or there is a lack of fluid replacement such as drinking water, dehydration can result.
- A dehydrated person stops sweating so evaporation is no longer effective in cooling the body. This can lead to heat exhaustion, the most severe of all heat-related disorders.
- The most important strategy to avoid, or at least minimize, the heat-related disorders of heat cramps, heat exhaustion, and heat stroke is frequent fluid replacement.
- The windchill factor—the combination of cold temperatures and windy conditions—presents the greatest danger for cold weather exercisers.

- In cold temperature, dehydration can be prevented by fluid replacement, and frostbite can be prevented by dressing in layers and wearing mittens and a woolen hat.
- Common causes of backaches are incorrect postures, improper exercises, and tight back and weak abdominal muscles, combined with short hamstring and hip flexor muscles.
- Physical activity (see the section Exercises for a Healthy Back) is one of the most prescribed strategies for preventing and treating back problems.
- Although participating in physical activities offers many benefits, it can also increase your risk for injuries.

- The four main causes of injuries are overuse, weakness and inflexibility, mechanical problems, and footwear.
- Prevention is the key to avoid, or at least minimize, the incidence of injuries. To prevent injuries, see table 9.6 in this chapter.
- Common injuries experienced by exercisers range from sprains and strains to tendinitis, bursitis, and muscle soreness.
- The R.I.C.E. formula is recommended for reducing the initial inflammation and alleviating pain (rest, ice, compression, and elevation).
- Many types of exercise should be avoided because they place excessive stresses, strains, or compression forces on particular muscles or joints.

A C T I V I T Y   9

EXERCISES FOR A HEALTHY BACK

Name _____   *To be submitted:*   *Yes*   *No*

Date _____   *If yes, due date* _____

Class _____   Section _____   Score _____

PURPOSE
To acquaint you with several exercises for developing and maintaining a healthy back.

DIRECTIONS
1. Follow the directions for the healthy back exercises found on pages 112 to 116.

2. Perform each exercise two to three times and hold each stretch for ten seconds.

3. If you have an existing back problem, check with your physician and inform your instructor before proceeding with this activity.

RESULTS
1. Did you enjoy performing the exercises for a healthy back?   Yes   No

2. Did you notice any difference with your back after completing the routine?   Yes   No   Explain.

3. To maintain a healthy back, what exercises do you think you would like to perform on a regular basis?

10

STRATEGIES TO STAY MOTIVATED TO EXERCISE

Motivational strategies—the key to staying fit year-round for your lifetime!

LEARNING OBJECTIVE

- Identify and describe several motivational strategies for exercise adherence.

LIFESTYLE QUESTIONS

- Have you ever been a regular exerciser, and then stopped and not started back up again? If yes, why did you stop exercising?

- If you are a regular exerciser, what motivates you to stay with it?

- If you're not a regular exerciser, what would motivate you to be a year-round exerciser?

INTRODUCTION

Sticking with a physical fitness program is **exercise adherence.** Have you ever wondered why some people stick with a year-round physical fitness program and others do not? Is there a magic formula for being a regular exerciser? No! However, to stay with a new behavior can be a challenge, especially if you plan to be a regular exerciser after years of being inactive. This is why adopting strategies to keep you motivated to exercise is so essential. Chapter 3 highlighted the steps to change health and fitness behavior. This chapter will be more specific in examining strategies you can use to stick with a year-round fitness program for a lifetime.

MOTIVATIONAL STRATEGIES

Believe in the Importance of Exercise

You must believe that there is a reason to keep exercising for you to continue doing it. A value that is based on sound knowledge can contribute to a strong motivation to continue. If you do believe that exer-

cise is important for you, you will likely stay with it. Those who are regular exercisers have a common belief that exercise is good for them.

Everything in life has a price. To continue any activity, you must believe that the benefits you receive from it are worth the price you will pay. To continue a regular fitness program, you must believe that the benefits you receive from it are worth your time, energy, and money.

Place Exercise as a High Priority

Regular exercise must be important enough to put into your regular schedule. If you place a high priority on your fitness program, you will fit it into your schedule. Don't let unimportant things interfere with your planned time to exercise. Make it a point to exercise at your scheduled time. Most people will respect you for sticking with your exercise commitment. Perhaps more important, you will have more respect for yourself.

Reach Your Goals

For some of us, the motivation to continue exercising comes from achievement. Set attainable goals for yourself. Then, when you reach them, you will feel a sense

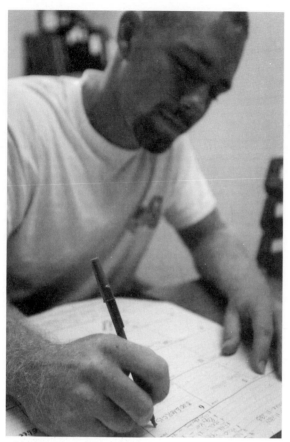

Blocking out time in your planner is a motivational strategy to exercise.

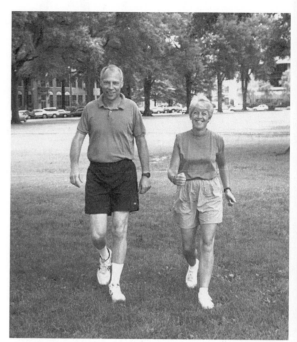

If you enjoy exercise, you will tend to stick with it.

of accomplishment. Some of your exercise goals should be related to exercise adherence. One of your greatest achievements could be a lifetime of regular exercise.

Make Time for Exercise

A common excuse given for not exercising is "I don't have time to exercise." We all have the same amount of time each day, each week, each month, and each year. You must decide what is most important in your life and schedule your time accordingly. If being fit is important to you, you will find time for it.

Enjoy Exercise

Enjoyment is important to exercise adherence. If exercise is fun, you are more likely to do it. You can find exercise enjoyment in many ways. Some factors that bring enjoyment during exercise are selecting a fun activity, competition, excitement, relaxation, social interaction, and challenge. What produces exercise enjoyment for you?

Make Exercise Convenient

Many people claim the reason they do not exercise is because it is too inconvenient. To combat this, make

your fitness program as convenient as possible. The more available exercise is to you, the more likely you are to stick with it. Here are some strategies to make exercise convenient for you:

- Consider taking an activity class at school.
- Locate a convenient location like your school's gym or nearby fitness center.
- Divide your exercise into smaller blocks of time, say for fifteen minutes twice a day or for ten minutes three times a day.
- Place your exercise shoes in a highly visible place.

Pace Yourself

If you are out of shape and want to get back in shape, take your time and pace yourself. Pushing too hard, especially when beginning a fitness program, can leave you frustrated, sore, and disinterested—exactly what you don't want! Slowly progress week by week by adding either small amounts of time, short distances, or small increases in intensity. This will help minimize soreness, bring positive results, and keep your motivation high for a lifelong fitness program.

Add Variety (Cross-Train)

Every day there are some people who are motivated in their fitness program to do the same exercise, at the same time, and at the same intensity. Others are motivated by doing different activities, at different times, and at different intensities every day. Adding variety or cross-training could include swimming Monday, Wednesday, and Friday and weight training

TABLE 10.1

Popular Activities and Their Important Considerations

Activity	Important Considerations
Walking, jogging, and running	* Use quality shoes * Walk, jog, or run facing traffic * At night, go with other people
Weight training	* Start out slowly and progress gradually * Consider enrolling in a weight-training class
Cycling	* Use a quality bicycle * Always wear a helmet * Pedal continuously * Ride with traffic
Stationary bicycling	* Use a quality bicycle * Add variety by reading a book, watching TV, etc. * Pedal continuously
Swimming	* Improve your skill level by taking lessons * Add different strokes for variety * Always swim with others or make sure a lifeguard is available
Dance, step, and water aerobics	* Go at your own pace * Use quality shoes * Make sure instructor is certified
Racquet sports (tennis, squash, racquetball)	* Use quality shoes and equipment * Pace yourself when first beginning the activity
Other sports (basketball, soccer, volleyball, golf, bowling, etc.)	* Don't overdo when first beginning the activity * Play continuously for optimal health benefits * Use quality shoes and equipment

on Tuesday, Thursday, and Saturday. Most of us like some change in our fitness program. To stay motivated and to prevent burnout and injury, consider adding variety to your fitness program. Table 10.1 presents many popular activities you can use to stick with a lifelong fitness program.

Tell Others

If you are starting an exercise program and think you might need support to stick with it, tell everyone you know. Most of us need the aid of our family and friends to stay with our goals. Once you have told others you are going to begin exercising, it is easier to stay with it.

Chart Your Progress

Record information about each of your exercise sessions in a consistent way. Some people use an exercise log, some use a notebook, some use a calendar, and some use a piece of paper to record their exercise accomplishments. There are many ways to do this, but somehow give yourself written credit for each exercise session.

Record information from your exercise session so you can visually see your successes accumulate. Soon you will have overwhelming evidence that you can stick with it.

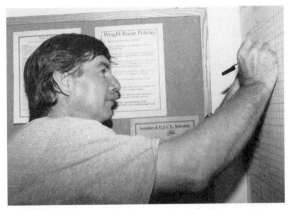

Documenting your performance will help you stay on task.

Reward Yourself

Regular exercisers seem to experience a sense of satisfaction—an intrinsic reward—from regular exercise. It makes them feel good. Extrinsic rewards such as clothing, new shoes, and money may help get a person to start a fitness program and stay motivated for a while. However, it is unlikely that these rewards will continue to motivate a person over a lifetime of exercise. Ultimately, if exercise does not make a person feel good, he or she will probably quit. On the

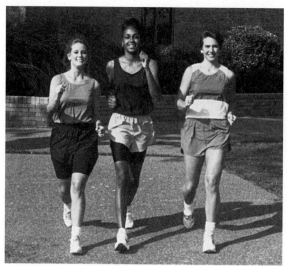

Exercising with others can serve as a powerful motivational strategy to maintain a fitness program.

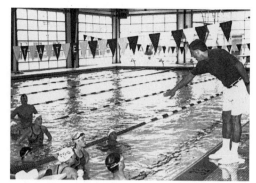

Taking lessons to raise your skill level will improve your performance and increase your enjoyment.

other hand, people who have an intrinsic reward system and feel good about their exercise program are much more likely to stick with it.

Exercise with Others

Many people enjoy social exercise. For them, exercising with others is a powerful motivation. Some like to exercise with one friend, whereas others like to exercise with a group. If you enjoy socializing while you exercise, build that into your plan. You may even enjoy participating in special exercise events with others, such as running or walking events. You might enjoy this for the competition, for the recognition, or for the opportunity to be with others who have similar values and beliefs about exercise.

Develop a History of Exercise Participation

As you develop a history of being a regular exerciser, it will become a part of your identity. Others will expect you to exercise. You will expect yourself to exercise.

Raise Your Skill Level

Most of us enjoy what we do well. If you are highly skilled at something, you probably enjoy it. Exercise is no exception. If you believe you are "good" at some activity, you are more likely to stick with it. To become "good" at an exercise activity, consider taking lessons. Receiving quality instruction when beginning an activity is an excellent investment of your time and money. Good lessons are generally a shortcut to better performance. Once you have learned the basic skills of an activity, it is important to continue

to practice. Find partners near or at your skill level so you can both enjoy the activity together. People with similar skill levels tend to motivate each other.

Keep a Balance Sheet

Some people are motivated by a balance sheet. An exercise balance sheet contains a list of your advantages and disadvantages for exercise. The balance sheet helps to keep a focus on your reasons to exercise. Whenever you are tempted to skip a workout, look at your list of advantages. This can provide an extra incentive to put on your exercise clothes and take the hardest step of all—the first one.

Strive for Success

Exercise adherence can give you a feeling of success. Since success breeds success, once you have experienced it with your fitness program, you are more likely to continue. Each of us can taste success at improving and maintaining fitness.

Form a Habit of Exercise

Optimal benefits of exercise come from many years of consistent participation. Regular exercise needs to become a lifestyle behavior. Like eating food and brushing teeth—it should be done on a daily basis throughout life.

SUMMARY

- Sticking with a physical fitness program is known as exercise adherence.
- There is no magic formula for being a regular exerciser. However, staying with a new behavior can be a challenge. This is especially true if you plan to be a regular exerciser after years of being inactive. This is why adopting strategies to keep you motivated to exercise is so essential.

- Motivational strategies for sticking with a fitness program include:
    1. Believe in the importance of exercise.
    2. Place exercise as a high priority.
    3. Reach your goals.
    4. Make time for exercise.
    5. Enjoy exercise.
    6. Make exercise convenient.
    7. Pace yourself.
    8. Add variety (cross-train).
    9. Tell others. Chart your progress.
    10. Reward yourself.
    11. Exercise with others.
    12. Develop a history of exercise participation.
    13. Raise your skill level.
    14. Keep a balance sheet.
    15. Strive for success.
    16. Form a habit of exercise.

A C T I V I T Y   10
THE EXERCISE ADHERENCE ASSESSMENT

Name _____   **To be submitted: Yes   No**

Date _____   **If yes, due date** _____

Class _____ **Section** _____   **Score** _____

PURPOSE
To assess your thoughts and attitudes about exercise and a lifelong fitness program.

DIRECTIONS
1. Read each of the questions in the Exercise Adherence Assessment and check either the yes, sometimes, or no column.

2. Answer the questions in the Results section.

EXERCISE ADHERENCE ASSESSMENT
1. Do you believe in the importance of exercise?	Yes	Sometimes	No
2. Do you have a positive attitude about exercise?	Yes	Sometimes	No
3. Do you place exercise as a high priority in your life?	Yes	Sometimes	No
4. Do you enjoy exercise?	Yes	Sometimes	No
5. Do you have fitness goals written down or clearly stated in your mind?	Yes	Sometimes	No
6. Do you like your current level of fitness?	Yes	Sometimes	No
7. Do you have a history of exercise participation?	Yes	Sometimes	No

RESULTS
1. What can you conclude from your answers to the assessment?

2. If you are a current exerciser, what motivational strategies do you use to stay with your program?

3. If you're not a current exerciser, what motivational strategies could you use from this chapter to start and stay with a fitness program?

CHAPTER 11

STRATEGIES TO BE A WISE HEALTH AND FITNESS CONSUMER

To protect your health and save your pocketbook, be a smart consumer!

LEARNING OBJECTIVES

- Discuss key concepts for being an intelligent consumer of fitness products and services.

- Describe the strategies for purchasing home exercise equipment available for use today.

- Identify key criteria for choosing a health/fitness club.

- Determine how reliable the sources are for health and fitness information.

LIFESTYLE QUESTIONS

- What fitness products (i.e., weights, bicycles, in-line skates) have you ever purchased to improve your level of fitness?

- What services, if any, have you used (i.e., massage therapists, personal trainers) to improve your level of fitness?

- What exercise equipment, if any, do you now use to improve your level of fitness?

- Do you belong to a health/fitness club or have friends who belong?

- Are you cautious about the health and fitness information you get from media sources such as television and radio?

- Are you cautious with what you read about health and fitness information from books and magazine articles?

INTRODUCTION

An explosion of health/fitness products and services has occurred in the last decade. One cannot turn around without noticing an unprecedented media advertising blitz. The stereotypical image of a healthy and fit body can be seen on numerous magazine covers in grocery stores, on television, and in newspaper ads. Advertised products and services include everything from home exercise equipment, weight loss pills, and health foods to fitness clubs and massage therapists.

Interest in health and fitness products and services is at an all-time high. Billions of dollars are spent each year on sporting goods and fitness equipment. For example, yearly sales of sporting goods are now over $20 billion, annual sales of athletic shoes and athletic clothing is at $2 and $4 billion, respectively, and sales of home equipment have jumped to $3 bil-

lion today. Sales of health foods, diet pills, hair-loss remedies, vitamins, and diet and exercise books continue to soar. And there is no end in sight. This is why, more than ever, we need to protect our health and our pocketbook by practicing **consumerism** (the ability to make intelligent decisions about health products and services).

THE INTELLIGENT CONSUMER

We as a society are more interested in health and fitness than ever before. However, it is essential that we become intelligent consumers of health products and services or risk adverse effects, including injury, illness, and money loss. There can be no debate that most, if not all, of us generally seek ways to remain youthful and attractive, to be fit and healthy, and to

TABLE 11.1

Strategies for Being an Intelligent Health/Fitness Consumer

1. **Become well informed by researching information and checking with reliable experts.** Becoming well informed takes considerable effort but is well worth the effort in the long run. Just as when you buy a major appliance, it is important to ask questions and do your homework by conducting a complete background check before buying or using a health/fitness product or service.

2. **Seek reliable sources of information.** Most reliable professionals include physicians, dentists, allied health professionals, health and fitness educators, and specialists in the health field. Federal, state, and local government; professionals; and voluntary agencies are generally also credible sources.

3. **Be skeptical about health and fitness information.** Develop a good pattern of not accepting statements at face value that appear in the news media or advertising. Ask questions about accuracy, scientific evidence, sources of information, qualifications of researcher(s), design of study, and so on.

4. **Check with others before buying.** Check with others who have already bought and/or used the same health and fitness product or service you are interested in. Also, find out who are the experts in this field and call them for their insight and advice.

5. **Check with the Better Business Bureau.** Call the Better Business Bureau to determine if any complaints have been filed against a company or center you are considering using a service of or buying a product from.

6. **Speak out!** Report any wrongdoing, quackery (questionable products or services), or fraud (where there is deliberate deception of a promoted, for-profit medical remedy known to be false or unproved).

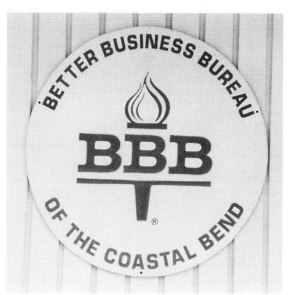

Check with the Better Business Bureau to determine if any complaints have been filed against a company you are considering doing business with.

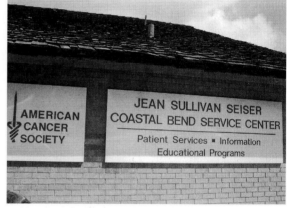

The American Cancer Society is a reputable organization that offers many educational and patient services.

fully enjoy the pleasures of living a productive and rewarding life. Many economic, social, and technological advances in achieving these goals have occurred. Due to these advancements, we have been led to believe that health, like any other item, can be purchased.

Many entrepreneurs, aware of consumers desires to purchase health and fitness quickly and easily, have flooded the market with ineffective or unsafe products and services to accommodate those who want a pleasurable and pain-free life. Also, the media, in an effort to earn high ratings and make money for their stockholders, have disseminated misinformation—ranging from the faintly biased to the downright wrong—to their gullible audience. It is no wonder we as consumers are confused by those who sell health products and services, and those who disseminate health information. This is why, more than ever, we need to adopt the philosophy, "let the seller beware," and become wise consumers.

Reading and understanding the information in this chapter will help you to make informed decisions about health and fitness products and services. Intelligent consumers have the knowledge and skills to research information and ask the right questions before purchas-

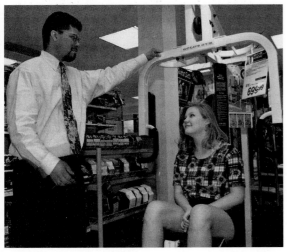

Make wise, informed decisions about the purchase and use of health products and services.

ing health products and services and believing everything they see or hear from the media. (See table 11.1.)

PURCHASING HOME FITNESS EQUIPMENT

Home exercise equipment is an industry that has become very lucrative. From treadmills to stairwalkers and from stationary exercise bikes to free weights and weight machines, home exercise equipment has become "in vogue." There is no debate that having exercise equipment at your residence allows you to exercise more conveniently. However, be forewarned about buying home exercise equipment. What often happens for many well-intentioned exercisers is this—the equipment is used for a short time before becoming a dust collector and adopted as a clothes hanger. The following strategies highlighted in table 11.2 are helpful in choosing home exercise equipment that can be used for a lifetime. It is advisable to start at a slow or moderate pace with limited duration and gradually increase over a period of time.

JOINING A HEALTH OR FITNESS CLUB

Joining a health or fitness club has become popular among many exercisers. These clubs offer many benefits to consumers, including qualified instruction, a variety of equipment, a supportive environment, and services such as fitness assessments, aerobic classes, and massage therapy. However, it is not nec-

TABLE 11.2
Strategies for Purchasing Home Exercise Equipment

1. **Check your commitment rating.** Make sure this piece of equipment is something you have wanted for a while and you are really committed to. Just because a friend recently purchased one or it's the latest craze in home exercise equipment will probably not be enough motivation to keep your commitment level high.

2. **There is no need to buy a lot of exercise equipment.** Unless you have lots of money or just enjoy collecting "stuff," keep in mind that a total physical fitness program can be carried out without any equipment.

3. **Write down your fitness goals you want to achieve using the new piece of exercise equipment.** Writing your goals will raise the likelihood that you will stay motivated to use the equipment.

4. **Try out the equipment more than once.** Sometimes exercisers are so excited the first time they use new equipment that they can't wait to buy it and take it home. Allowing some time after trying it out will help ensure your interest remains high.

5. **Buy from a well-established, reputable company that will back up its warranties.** Some companies are here one day, gone the next. When possible, avoid mail-order products because it may be difficult to make an exchange or return the item(s).

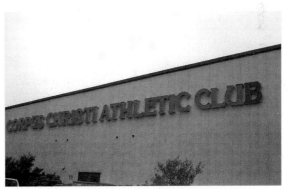

Make sure your commitment level is high, and ask lots of questions before joining a fitness club.

essary to join a private club to improve your health and fitness. Chances are your college or local Y offers similar equipment and services for a less expensive price and without long-term contracts. If joining a private club is for you, consider the following strategies found in table 11.3.

TABLE 11.3

Strategies to Use Before Joining a Club

1. Check the club's reputation with the Better Business Bureau and see if any complaints have been registered.

2. If possible, choose a no-contract, pay-as-you-go setup. This way, if you decide to stop attending, you won't lose any money like you would with a contract.

3. Ask whether a trial membership is possible to see if you like the environment.

4. **Before signing a contract,** do some careful questioning. Find out how long the club has been in existence, contact some club members for their observations, and request a complete tour of the facility.

5. Thoroughly check out the qualifications of the club's personnel. Do they have a background in physical education, kinesiology, or exercise physiology? Are they certified by the American College of Sports Medicine as exercise leaders, health/fitness instructors, or exercise specialists? Are the personal trainers and aerobics instructors certified?

6. Make certain you read and understand every word of the contract. If a section is unclear, consult with an attorney.

7. Make sure the location of the club is close or easily accessible.

8. Attend the club at the hours you are most likely to go. This way, you will discover what the traffic getting there and leaving there is like, if it is overcrowded, if equipment is available, if there is assistance if you need it, and if you would enjoy the type of people who are already members.

9. Be cautious about accepting diets, drugs, or food supplements from the club. Your physician will prescribe these if he or she feels they would be helpful to you.

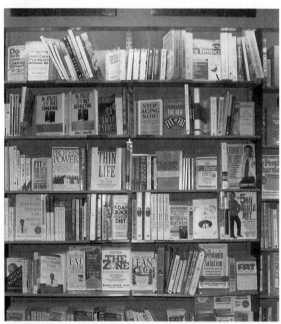

There are numerous health and fitness books on the market.

CHOOSING RELIABLE HEALTH/FITNESS MAGAZINES, BOOKS, AND ARTICLES

Publishers are motivated by profit, and since publishing is a highly competitive and lucrative field, selection of material is often based on what sells the best. Publishers know that the more popular, fa-

mous, or attractive the authors are, or the more sensational or different their ideas are, the better chance for that magazine or book to sell. Want to become rich and famous? As the joke goes, write a diet book! You often find movie stars, models, TV personalities, and even Olympic athletes as the authors of health/fitness books and articles; yet these individuals are rarely trained in academic fields that would qualify them as experts in advising others on fitness and health matters.

Most people in the United States learn the majority of their health and fitness information by reading books and popular magazines. Go to a bookstore and an entire section is usually devoted to health and fitness books. Pick up a popular magazine and you'll probably find at least one article dealing with health and fitness. Some of the authors of these health and fitness publications are experts in their respective fields. Some are simply professional writers who have interviewed these experts. Others have celebrity status who are attractive and look fit. Of these celebrities, some have written excellent books and articles supported and documented by reliable and current information. However, too many others have publications that contain misinformation.

Unreliable health and fitness information not based on the scientific method of controlled experimentation can lead to major disappointment and failure, and can contribute to poor health in those who follow the ill-fated advice. Common examples of publications with unreliable information are books

TABLE 11.4

Strategies to Evaluate Reliable Sources of Health and Fitness Information

1. Check out the author. Is the author an expert in the field? Does he or she have a degree or adequate training in this field the book or article is written in?

2. Check out the source of the publication. Is the book or magazine publisher credible?

3. Is the book or article up-to-date?

4. Does the book or magazine article refrain from using terms such as quick, miraculous, easy, new discovery, remove fat, or any other misleading words?

5. Does the information contained in the book or article appear reliable, practical, and achievable?

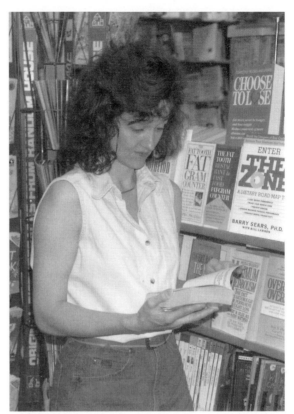

Before buying, make sure the information in the book or article is reliable, practical, and achievable.

on diets that promise to take fifteen pounds off in two weeks and articles on exercise workouts that claim consumers only need to exercise a few minutes twice a week to attain complete fitness. Check the strategies in table 11.4 to evaluate reliable sources of health and fitness information.

SUMMARY

- An explosion for health and fitness products and services has occurred in the last decade. Interest is at an all-time high in health and fitness as demonstrated by the billions of dollars spent on sporting goods and exercise equipment.
- Consumerism is the ability to make intelligent decisions about health products and services.
- Being unwise consumers can lead to adverse effects including injury, illness, and money loss.
- Many people believe that health is purchasable. Entrepreneurs capitalize on consumers' desires to purchase health and fitness quickly and easily, by flooding the market with products and services that are unsafe or ineffective.
- The media also plays a major role with health and fitness advertisements. The public can be deceived when misinformation is disseminated by the media.
- An intelligent consumer will have the knowledge and skills to research information and ask the right questions before purchasing health and fitness products and services.
- Strategies for being an intelligent fitness/health consumer include: be well-informed by researching information and checking with experts, seek

reliable sources of information, be skeptical about health and fitness information, check with others before buying, check with the Better Business Bureau (BBB), and speak out about any wrongdoing, quackery, or fraud.
- The home exercise equipment industry has become very lucrative. However, although it has become popular to own home equipment, be forewarned that without commitment, interest will fade and equipment will become unused.
- Strategies for purchasing home exercise equipment include: check your commitment level; do not buy a lot of exercise equipment; write down your goals before purchasing any equipment; try the equipment more than once; and buy from a well-established and reputable company that will back up its warranties.
- Joining a health or fitness club has become popular among many exercisers. However, it is not necessary to join a club to improve your health and fitness. The local Y or your college probably offers similar equipment and services as a private club.
- Strategies to remember before joining a club can be found in table 11.3.

- Most people in the United States learn the majority of their health and fitness information by reading books and popular magazines.
- Unreliable health and fitness information not based on the scientific method of controlled experimentation can lead to major disappointment and failure and can contribute to poor health in those who follow ill-fated advice.
- Strategies to evaluate reliable sources of health and fitness information include: check out the author; check out the source of the publication; note whether the article or book is current; determine whether the article or book refrains from using terms such as quick, miraculous, easy, new discovery, remove fat, or any other misleading words; and assess whether the information contained in the book or article appears sensible, practical, and attainable.

A C T I V I T Y   **11**

BE A WISE HEALTH CONSUMER!

Name _____   *To be submitted:*   *Yes*   *No*

Date _____   *If yes, due date* _____

Class _____   Section _____   *Score* _____

PURPOSE
To become an intelligent consumer of health and fitness products and services.

DIRECTIONS
1. Visit a store that sells home exercise equipment. Interview an employee working in the exercise equipment department by asking him or her the questions located in the Results section. Write the employee's responses in the spaces provided.

2. Visit a health or fitness club. Interview an employee by asking him or her the questions located in the Results section. Write the responses in the spaces provided.

3. Visit a bookstore. Evaluate a book and magazine article in health and fitness that you have an interest in. Answer the questions located in the Results section.

RESULTS

Home Exercise Equipment Interview

1. How long has this store been here?

2. How is business at your store with home exercise equipment?

3. What pieces of equipment are most popular?

4. What pieces of equipment are least popular?

5. How do you like working here?

6. What is your warranty on your most expensive pieces of exercise equipment?

Health or Fitness Club Interview

1. How long has this club been here?

2. Approximately how many members belong here?

3. What services do you provide here (fitness assessments, aerobics, massage, tennis and swimming lessons, etc.)?

4. What are the qualifications of the personnel who work here?

5. Do you have a pay-as-you-go plan or trial membership option?

6. Describe your contract for new members.

7. What are your hours?

8. Does your club offer a weight loss program where food supplements, drugs, or pills are prescribed?

9. How do you like working here?

Evaluating Books, Magazines, and Articles

1. Are the authors of the book and magazine article you evaluated experts in this particular field? What qualifications and training do they have?

2. What was the subject of the book? The magazine article?

3. Does the book or magazine's cover contain any terms such as quick, miraculous, easy, new discovery, remove fat, or any other misleading words? If yes, which ones?

4. After skimming through the book and magazine article, did the information appear to be based on scientific study?

3

OTHER STRATEGIES FOR WELLNESS

12

STRATEGIES FOR HEALTHY NUTRITION

Balance, variety, and moderation—the formula for healthy eating!

LEARNING OBJECTIVES

- Define nutrition and understand its relationship to wellness.

- Discuss the importance of balance, variety, and moderation for healthy nutrition.

- Identify and describe the six classes of nutrients.

- Explain the Food Guide Pyramid and the Dietary Guidelines for Americans.

- Interpret the 80/20 rule for healthy nutrition.

- Investigate the concerns about fast foods.

- Discuss how to read labels.

- Identify foods recommended for good health by dietitians.

LIFESTYLE QUESTIONS

- Would you describe your eating patterns as nutritious?

- Do you mainly consume healthy or unhealthy snacks?

- Do you mainly consume healthy or unhealthy liquids?

- Do you like fruits and vegetables?

- Do you know how much fat you are consuming in your diet?

- Do you often eat a lot of fast foods?

- Do you usually read food labels?

INTRODUCTION

Each day we have many choices to make about food: when to eat, what to eat, and how much to eat. We also all have to eat and drink to stay alive. This is one lifestyle behavior that is mandatory. The key is to eat and drink for energy and health, not just because food tastes good or is convenient. Experts are in agreement that our eating patterns play a major role in our level of well-being.

Nutrition experts agree that healthy nutrition is built on balance, variety, and moderation. This means enjoying many different foods in moderate portions, without having to give up your favorite selections. A healthy diet can prevent the consumption of too many calories, too much of any one nutrient, or too much of any single food.

The college years often bring about changes in food patterns. Factors such as class attendance, long study hours, work, finances, and extracurricular activities can interfere with normal eating patterns. As a result of busy schedules, college students become more dependent on fast foods, delivery services, and vending machines to satisfy appetite and supply energy to the body.

WHAT IS NUTRITION?

Nutrition comes from the Latin word that means "to nourish," or to provide all that is necessary to sustain life. **Human nutrition, therefore, is defined as the science of food, the study of its uses within the body, and its relationship to health.** Proper nutrition sustains life by promoting good health. The

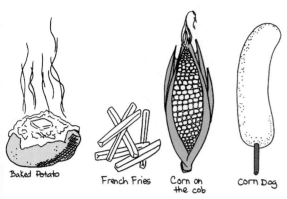

What are your choices?

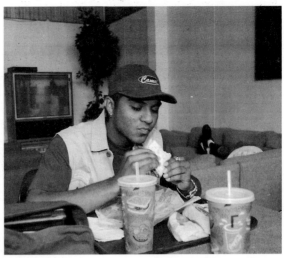

Is your selection of foods and drinks mainly healthy or unhealthy?

study of nutrition involves knowing about approximately forty-six essential nutrients, which fall into six major categories: **carbohydrates, proteins, fats, vitamins, minerals, and water.** Nutrition is concerned with how the body utilizes these nutrients and their effects on your health. Finally, positive nutritional behavior includes choosing the daily recommended servings from the Food Guide Pyramid and following the dietary guidelines recommended for Americans by the U.S. Department of Agriculture.

NUTRITION AND WELLNESS

Proper nutrition has long been considered an important factor contributing to a healthy lifestyle. With overwhelming evidence from research studies that shows connections between diet and health, interest in nutrition has soared. Positive nutritional practices can enhance growth, development, and optimal health. In addition, eating well can improve vitality, enhance quality of life, and lead to greater life expectancy. On the other hand, unhealthy nutritional behaviors, such as high-fat diets, can be a contributing factor to such problems as heart disease, cancer, stroke, diabetes, obesity, gallstones, and arthritis.

Although the act of eating is a voluntary activity, it becomes habitual because it is given hardly any thought. More than a thousand times a year, you choose to eat a meal. In your lifetime, you will consume more than seventy thousand meals. Imagine how many thousands of pounds of food that is! In one day, your eating selections may affect your health only slightly, but in the long term they become cumulative.

Most people need to distinguish between **hunger** and **appetite.** *Hunger* is the physiological need for food; *appetite* is the desire to eat. Your body's physiological need for food is often satisfied much sooner than is your appetite. To promote good health, we need to learn to control appetite. There is, indeed, some truth in the saying, "Always leave the table a little hungry."

Food affects all dimensions of wellness. Most people view food as only affecting the physical dimension of wellness, when actually it influences all dimensions (see fig. 12.1). To a large degree, our social dimension is centered around food, not around nutrition. For example, the good host offers guests something to eat and drink, because what would a party or casual get-together be like without food or drink? Food can be used also to comfort us emotionally when we're sad or upset, or it can be used as a reward during happy times. These are but a few examples of the importance of food in society.

CALORIES (KILOCALORIES)

The term **Calorie** is used to indicate the energy-producing value of food when oxidized in the body. When discussing nutrition, we use *Calorie* (with a capital C), which is actually a **kilocalorie (kcal)** and is defined as the amount of heat (or energy) required to raise the temperature of 1 *kilogram* (or 1,000 grams) of water by 1 degree Celsius. If an apple, therefore, contains a hundred Calories, it provides a hundred units of energy. See table 12.1 for the caloric values of nutrients and how they apply to each nutrient.

THE SIX CLASSES OF NUTRIENTS

The six classes of nutrients are carbohydrates, fats, proteins, vitamins, minerals, and water (see fig. 12.2). Basically, nutrients perform three functions.

FIGURE 12.1
Food Affects all Wellness Components

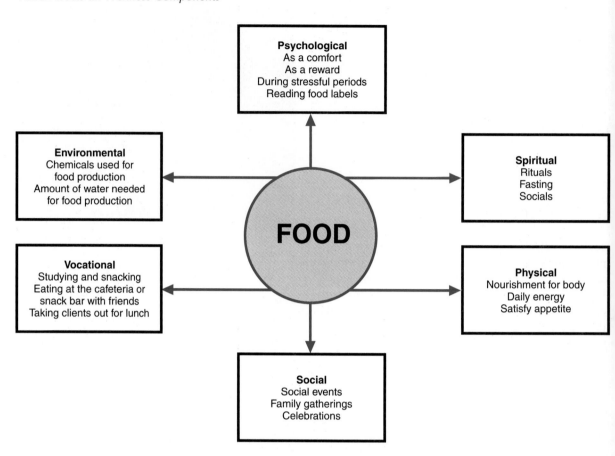

First, nutrients such as carbohydrates, fats, and proteins provide energy for the body. Protein's major function, however, is to build and repair tissue rather than be used as a major source of energy. Second, protein and certain minerals, such as calcium, are nutrients that help build and maintain body tissue. Finally, nutrients such as protein, vitamins, minerals, and water help regulate body functions; for example, oxygen attaches to the iron molecules of hemoglobin and is carried to the body's cells.

Carbohydrates

The ideal fuel source for the body, carbohydrates contribute to about half of the body's energy needs, without which no other metabolic activity could occur. They do so in the form of glucose, a sugar into which all carbohydrates eventually break down. In fact, *glucose* is the most important sugar for the cells of the human body.

There are two major types of carbohydrates. The first is called **complex carbohydrates.** They are made up of starches, in which form they are the easiest nutrients for the body to digest, absorb, and utilize. Because of this, starches are the staple food for most of the

world. Foods such as pasta, rice, whole-grain breads, cereals, and starchy vegetables such as corn, potatoes, and winter squash provide rich sources of carbohydrates. Besides providing long-term, or sustained, energy, these complex carbohydrates also supply the body with other desirable nutrients, including water, protein, fiber, vitamins, and minerals.

The second type of carbohydrate is labeled **simple** because of its molecular structure. These are the sugars, which also provide energy to the body, but for a shorter period of time than do the starches. In fact, all carbohydrates, simple and complex, are changed into **glucose** before being used as energy by the body. Other sugars in our diet include **fructose** (found in fruits, honey, and maple syrup), **sucrose** (table sugar), and **lactose** (milk sugar), which comes mainly from milk.

Fiber, a carbohydrate, is associated with many health benefits, even though it contains no Calories or energy for the body. Known also as roughage and bulk, fiber is made up of indigestible carbohydrates that pass through the digestive tract without being absorbed. We are not able to digest fiber because the body lacks an enzyme to break it

TABLE 12.1
The Caloric Value of Nutrients

Nutrient	Calories
1 gram of protein	4
1 gram of carbohydrates (sugar or starch)	4
1 gram of alcohol	7
1 gram of fat	9
Vitamins, minerals, water, fiber	0

How to Apply the Caloric Value to Each Nutrient

A serving of microwave popping corn (3 cups popped) contains 17 grams of carbohydrate, 3 grams of protein, 8 grams of fat, and 152 calories.

Carbohydrate:

17 grams × 4 calories per gram = calories from carbohydrate (68 ÷ 152 = 45%)

Protein:

3 grams × 4 calories per gram = 12 calories from protein (12 ÷ 152 = 8%)

Fat:

8 grams × 9 calories per gram = 72 calories from fat (72 ÷ 152 = 47%)
1 serving of microwave popping corn = 152 calories (45% carbohydrates, 8% proteins, and 47% fat)

FIGURE 12.2
The Six Classes of Nutrients Needed for Wellness

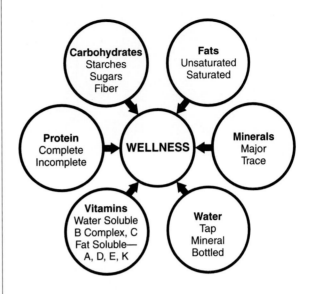

TABLE 12.2
Possible Health Benefits of Fiber

Fiber Type	Source	Possible Benefits
Insoluble	Brown rice	Promotes regularity
	Dried beans	Protects against colon cancer
	Fruits	Prevents obesity by replacing dietary fat
	Popcorn	Manages blood sugar
	Rye	
	Seeds	
	Vegetables	
	Wheat bran	
	Whole grains	
Soluble	Barley	Lowers blood cholesterol
	Dried beans	Manages blood sugar
	Fruits	Prevents obesity by replacing dietary fat
	Oat bran	
	Oatmeal	
	Rye	
	Seeds	
	Vegetables	

down. Table 12.2 highlights the two types of fiber, along with their sources and possible health benefits.

With a well-balanced diet, you are likely to get the different types of fiber and all their benefits. To consume enough fiber to enhance your health (25–35 grams daily), eat a well-balanced diet, making sure you consume ample amounts of whole grains, fruits, and vegetables daily. Some benefits from a high-fiber diet may actually come from the food containing the fiber, not from the fiber alone. Thus, it's better to receive fiber from foods rather than from supplements. To prevent intestinal problems such as bloating and gas, experts recommend increasing fiber gradually in the diet while drinking plenty of water.

Fats

A small amount of fat is required for good health. **Fats** (also known as **lipids**) provide energy; carry the fat-soluble vitamins A, D, E, and K in the blood; provide essential fatty acids needed for growth; insulate the body; are essential parts of every cell; and contribute to hormone synthesis and the blood-clotting mechanism. Unfortunately, people of all ages take in too much fat, leading to serious health problems.

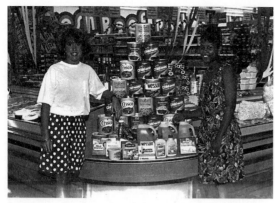

The average American adult consumes 115 pounds of fat per year.

TABLE 12.3
Strategies for Reducing Dietary Fat

1. Consume more grains, vegetables, and fruits.
2. Stick to recommended servings for meats (2–3 servings daily).
3. Substitute skim milk for whole milk.
4. Remove chicken skin before cooking or eating.
5. Substitute low-fat yogurt or sherbet for ice cream.
6. Purchase only lean meat cuts and trim visible fats.
7. Grill, bake, or broil instead of frying.
8. Use egg whites and limit egg yolks.
9. Limit salad dressing.
10. Limit high-fat snacks and desserts.
11. Have meatless meals once or twice a week.

Health experts recommend that people, especially those at risk for heart disease, eat less fat. It is recommended that **no more than 30 percent** of your Calories should come from fat, of which **no more than 10 percent** come from saturated fat choices (i.e., meats, milk, and milk products).

There are two types of fats in foods—saturated and unsaturated. Saturated fats, except for the tropical oils, come from animal sources and are usually solid at room temperature. It is this type of fat that is associated with heart disease and cancer of the breast, colon, and prostate. Saturated fats are found in meats, butter, milk, and in the tropical oils: palm, palm kernel, and coconut.

Unsaturated fats are found in plant sources and are liquid at room temperature. Two classes of unsaturated fats are **polyunsaturated** (corn, safflower, sesame, soybean, sunflower, and cottonseed oils) and **monounsaturated** (olive, peanut, and canola oils). Recent research shows that polyunsaturated fats aren't so healthy either because they lower the "good" **high-density lipoprotein (HDL)** cholesterol and may increase risk for certain types of cancer. This leaves monounsaturated oils as the fat of choice. They have been shown to lower the "bad" **low-density lipoprotein (LDL)** cholesterol but maintain the HDL cholesterol levels.

Cholesterol is a waxy, fatlike substance that is essential for life. Cholesterol is used to form cell membranes, the sex hormones estrogen and progesterone, and other vital substances. Cholesterol also ensures proper functioning of the nervous system. It is not a required nutrient because the body manufactures all the cholesterol it needs. Excess dietary cholesterol is linked to heart disease and strokes. Cholesterol is found in all animal foods, including meat, eggs, fish, poultry, and dairy products.

Cholesterol is carried in the bloodstream by LDLs and HDLs. The LDLs are believed to deposit cholesterol on artery walls, potentially causing coronary heart disease. HDLs are thought to carry cholesterol away from the cells in the arteries and transport it back to the liver for processing or removal.

Other studies have shown that the most significant factor in food that affects blood cholesterol is saturated fat in the diet, rather than dietary cholesterol. When saturated fat is introduced into the body (via diet), the liver produces cholesterol, thus raising both fat and cholesterol in the blood. These studies suggest reducing total fat in the diet and exercising to lower risk of heart disease (see table 12.3).

About half of all adults have cholesterol levels that are too high. An estimated 25 percent of all Americans have high cholesterol and another 25 percent are borderline-high. Have you had your blood cholesterol levels checked recently? If not, make an appointment with your physician. Ask to receive a complete "lipid profile," which includes total cholesterol, LDL, HDL, a ratio of total cholesterol to HDL, and triglycerides.

Olestra, a synthetic fat substitute, has been approved by the Food and Drug Administration to meet the increasing demand for low-fat, healthier processed foods. Although foods made with and cooked in Olestra are without the fat and Calories of the real nutrient, red flags are being raised by organizations such as the Center for Science in the Public Interest. They cite indications that Olestra can cause digestive dysfunction and may decrease the absorption of fat-soluble vitamins and carotenoids. To counteract some of the concerns regarding vitamin absorption, Procter & Gamble, the maker of Olestra, has added fat-soluble vitamins to its Olestra-containing products. Also, the company firmly believes that all questions as to the safety of Olestra have been answered by animal studies and clinical trials.

Protein

Protein is needed for growth, repair, and maintenance of all body cells. Protein also transmits hereditary characteristics and helps form the hormones and enzymes used to regulate body processes. Protein can be found in animal sources (meat, eggs, fish, and dairy products) and plant sources (dried beans and peas, whole grains, pasta, rice, and seeds).

Protein is made up of twenty different amino acids—the building blocks of the body. It is essential that nine of the amino acids be included in your diet, because your body cannot produce them. These nine essential amino acids must be present during the same meal for growth and repair of tissue to occur. The other eleven amino acids will be produced by the body. All twenty amino acids must be present in your body at the same time to form protein.

The two types of protein are called complete and incomplete. *Complete* protein comes from animal sources and contains all nine of the essential amino acids. One way to get all the amino acids you need is to include foods from animal sources in your daily diet. *Incomplete* protein comes from plant foods (vegetables and grains) and lacks one or more of the essential amino acids. If you do not eat meat products, you can still form complete protein by combining plant proteins with each other or with animal protein. Common examples of combining proteins include cereal and milk, rice and beans, macaroni and cheese, and peanut butter and jelly on whole-wheat bread.

Most Americans take in more protein than necessary for good health. Your daily protein requirements are 0.8 grams per kilogram (2.2 pounds) of body weight. This amounts to no more than 12 to 15 percent of your total daily Calories. A simple way to get a rough estimate of your protein needs is to take your weight and divide by three. If you weigh 150 pounds, your approximate daily protein needs would be 50 grams.

Vitamins

Vitamins are organic substances needed by the body in trace amounts. Vitamins work by enhancing the action of enzymes in the body, which enables us to use other nutrients. There are thirteen known vitamins, each responsible for performing a variety of specific and unique roles within the body. Vitamins help regulate important bodily functions such as manufacturing healthy blood cells and liberating energy from carbohydrates, fats, and proteins.

The two types of vitamins are water-soluble and fat-soluble. The vitamin B complex and vitamin C can be dissolved in water (water-soluble) and are more readily eliminated from the body. Vitamins A,

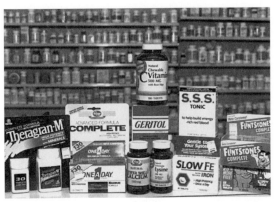

Vitamin supplementation becomes necessary if you are not following a well-balanced diet.

D, E, and K are transported, absorbed, and stored with body fat (fat-soluble). Since fat-soluble vitamins are not quickly eliminated, excessive amounts can lead to toxic, health-threatening effects. It should be noted that recent research has shown that megadosing with certain water-soluble vitamins have also resulted in side effects.

Most people do not need vitamin supplements. By eating a well-balanced and varied diet, you are likely to receive all the vitamins your body needs. In addition, many of our foods have been enriched and fortified, thus eliminating the need for vitamin supplementation. If you decide to take a vitamin supplement, choose a multiple vitamin that does not exceed 100 percent of the RDA. Anything above the RDA is a waste of money. In addition, there is no need to take the supplement every day because you are receiving vitamins from the food you eat. You may want to take the multiple vitamin every second or third day.

Certain people can benefit from taking vitamin supplements. Vegetarians, pregnant or breast-feeding women, women with excessive menstrual bleeding, strict dieters, and those not following a well-balanced diet should check with their physician about vitamin and mineral supplementation. In addition, those suffering from long-term illness and disease or taking medication that reduces appetite or hinders the body's ability to use nutrients should consult with their physicians.

Folic acid, a B vitamin, has become increasingly important in our diet to help prevent birth defects along with heart disease and stroke. Research has documented the importance for all women of childbearing age and those individuals with risk factors for health disease and stroke to consume 400 micrograms of folic acid (the Recommended Dietary Allowance) every day either through diet or supplementation. Because of its increasing importance, the

TABLE 12.4

Good Sources of Folic Acid

Food	Folic Acid (micrograms)
Total cereal (¾ cup)	400
Lentils (½ cup, cooked)	179
Pinto beans (½ cup, cooked)	145
Chickpeas (½ cup, cooked)	145
Spinach (½ cup, cooked)	131
Kidney beans (½ cup, cooked)	115
Orange juice (1 cup, from concentrate)	109
Spinach (1 cup, raw)	109
Most breakfast cereals (1 cup)	100
Romaine lettuce (1 cup, shredded)	76
Split peas (½ cup, cooked)	64
Broccoli (½ cup, cooked)	39

Source: USDA Handbook 8

FDA is considering fortification of folic acid to flour. This, in turn, would fortify such products as breads, pasta, and cereals. In the meantime, consume foods from table 12.4 or consider supplementation.

THE ANTIOXIDANT SUPPLEMENT DEBATE

The antioxidants of vitamin C, vitamin E, and beta-carotene have developed a reputation for their ability to protect us against our natural oxidative processes and ravages of the environment. Due to breathing and the normal oxidation of our cells, the body constantly produces reactive chemicals called **free radicals.** During vigorous exercise, the rate of production for free radicals increases and the body also acquires them from environmental sources such as cigarette smoke and air pollution. The problem with free radicals? They are unstable and wreak havoc on our stable cells. The damage caused by free radicals is believed to contribute to such conditions as heart disease, cancer, and aging. Antioxidants may protect the body from this damage by neutralizing the free radicals. Numerous studies have indicated that people who consume a diet high in antioxidant fruits and vegetables are less likely to develop diseases related to free radicals.

The jury is still out, however, on supplements. Conflicting study results have led some to abandon antioxidants because they can often act as pro-oxidants in supplements, boosting oxidant and free-radical production. Others, notably Dr. Kenneth Cooper, the highly respected father of the aerobics movement, claim we need them more than ever, especially if we enjoy vigorous exercise. Although further research is needed, it is safe to suggest that you should eat plenty of antioxidant-rich foods (see table 12.5). If you still feel you are not getting enough antioxidants from food, take a supplement, but do so in moderation.

Minerals

Minerals perform many vital functions in the body. From building strong bones and teeth (calcium) to forming hemoglobin in red blood cells (iron), minerals are essential for good nutrition. Like vitamins, minerals are needed in small amounts and do not supply energy. Other important functions include assisting in nerve transmission and muscle contraction, and regulating fluid levels and the acid-base balance of the body. Minerals can also be toxic in excess amounts. In the adult diet, mineral concerns include too much sodium and, for women, too little iron and calcium.

Minerals are classified into two types: major and trace. Calcium, sodium, phosphorous, chloride, potassium, and magnesium are considered major minerals because **they are needed in amounts greater than a hundred milligrams per day.** Trace minerals such as iron, zinc, iodine, selenium, and copper are needed only in tiny amounts. Because minerals are absorbed, utilized, and eliminated by the body, it is important to replace them on a daily basis. Eating a wide variety of nutritious foods is the best way to obtain sufficient quantities of the essential minerals. Fruits and vegetables are ideal mineral sources.

Water

Water is often called the "forgotten nutrient." Water may well be our most important nutrient because without it we would not live more than a week. More than half our body weight comes from water. Water provides the medium for nutrient and waste transportation and plays a vital role in nearly all our body's biochemical reactions. People seldom think about the importance of an adequate daily intake of water.

The average American drinks more soft drinks in a year than water. Adults require eight glasses of water a day, and even more with an active lifestyle. If you eat more fresh fruits and vegetables, you will require less water. Three sound recommendations for drinking more water include keeping a container of water in the refrigerator, drinking water throughout the day, and drinking water instead of beverages

TABLE 12.5

Selected Foods That Contain Antioxidants

Vitamin C	Vitamin E	Carotenoids (Beta-Carotene)	Mixed Antioxidants
Cabbage	Almonds	Apricots	Bran wheat
Cauliflower	Chick peas	Broccoli	Cloves
Grapefruit	Eggs	Cantaloupe	Green tea
Oranges	Hazelnuts	Carrots	Nutmeg
Peppers	Oatmeal	Kale	Pepper
Potatoes	Rye flour	Mustard greens	Rice
Raspberries	Soybeans	Spinach	Sesame
Strawberries	Sunflower seeds	Sweet potatoes	Thyme
Tangerines	Wheat germ	Winter squash	

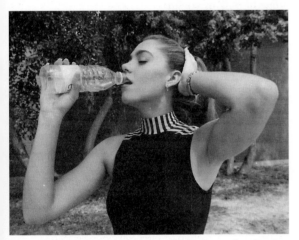

Carry a water bottle with you throughout the day in order to drink more water.

when dining out. Good choices are plain water from the tap and any kind of mineral water or bottled water. Many people put lemon or lime in their water to give it added flavor. Sweetened drinks (fruit drinks, soda), coffee, tea, and alcohol should be limited. Caffeine and alcohol speed up the effect of dehydration and necessitate an increase in water intake.

THE FOOD GUIDE PYRAMID

The U.S. Departments of Agriculture and Health and Human Services have recently adopted the Food Guide Pyramid, which replaces the Basic Four Food Groups. The new Food Guide Pyramid can help you choose the recommended servings from healthy foods to get the nutrients you need without excess calories, fats, cholesterol, sugar, or sodium.

The Food Guide Pyramid provides a simple, practical guide for general meal planning and can be used to evaluate your overall food intake pattern. The pyramid illustrates the five food groups with recommended servings that are important to a healthy diet (see fig. 12.3). The new diagram places the bread, cereal, rice, and pasta group at the base, taking up the largest section. Because it is rich in complex carbohydrates this group serves as the foundation of the diet. Vegetables and fruits are two equal groups instead of one and have the next largest sections. Above them as the pyramid narrows, meats and dairy products share a band. **At the top are fats, oils, and sweets, which are considered a food category rather than a food group.** This category is the smallest and should provide the fewest Calories.

DIETARY GUIDELINES FOR AMERICANS

The U.S. Departments of Agriculture and Health and Human Services have issued a recent report stating the revised set of dietary guidelines that promote realistically attainable health and dietary goals. The new guidelines promote moderation and include eating a wide variety of foods, balancing the foods we eat with physical activity, and using good judgment in our use of sugar, salt, and alcohol.

In the report, vegetarian diets were given attention for the first time. It stated that a good diet can exclude animal products like meat and milk but encouraged vegetarians to take vitamin B_{12} supplements and to find good sources of vitamin D and calcium. Also, the report recognized recent scientific discoveries,

FIGURE 12.3
Food Guide Pyramid

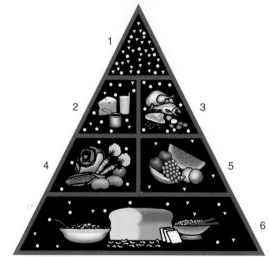

A Guide to Daily Food Choices

Source: U.S. Department of Agriculture/U.S. Department of Health and Human Services.

1. Fats, Oils, and Sweets
   USE SPARINGLY

2. Milk, Yogurt, and Cheese Group
   2–3 SERVINGS

3. Meat, Poultry, Fish,
   Dry Beans, Eggs,
   and Nuts Group
   2–3 SERVINGS

4. Vegetable Group
   3–5 SERVINGS

5. Fruit Group
   2–4 SERVINGS

6. Bread, Cereal, Rice,
   and Pasta Group
   6–11 SERVINGS

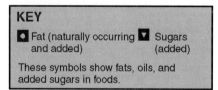

KEY

◆ Fat (naturally occurring ▼ Sugars
   and added)   (added)

These symbols show fats, oils, and
added sugars in foods.

How to Use the Daily Food Guide

What Counts as One Serving?

Breads, Cereals, Rice, and Pasta
1 slice of bread
½ cup of cooked rice or pasta
½ cup of cooked cereal
1 ounce of ready-to-eat cereal

Vegetables
½ cup of chopped raw or cooked vegetables
1 cup of leafy raw vegetables

Fruits
1 piece of fruit or melon wedge
¾ cup of juice
½ cup of canned fruit
¼ cup of dried fruit

Milk, Yogurt, and Cheese
1 cup of milk or yogurt
1½ to 2 ounces of cheese

Meat, Poultry, Fish, Dry Beans, Eggs, and Nuts
2½ to 3 ounces of cooked lean meat, poultry, or fish
   Count ½ cup of cooked beans, or 1 egg, or 2 table-
spoons of peanut butter as 1 ounce of lean meat
(about ⅓ serving)

Fats, Oils, and Sweets
Limit calories from these, especially if you need to
lose weight

> The amount you eat may be more than one
> serving. For example, a dinner portion of spaghetti
> would count as two or three servings of pasta.

Source: FDA Consumer, June 1993.

such as the health benefit of moderate alcohol consumption and a pregnant woman's need for folic acid
in her diet. The following are the new National
Health and Nutritional Guidelines:

Varied Diet: Eat grains, vegetables, fruit; choose
a diet low in fats and cholesterol; and watch intake of
salt, sodium and sugar.

Exercise: 30 minutes or more of moderate exercise in most days of the week.

Weight Maintenance: Weight should fall within
a given range according to height (see chapter 8,
table 8.4); weight loss should occur gradually.

Alcohol: Drink in moderation, with meals, and
when consumption does not put you or others at risk.

THE 80/20 RULE

*Another guide to follow for healthy nutrition is the
80/20 rule.* The 80/20 rule states that if you eat a
variety of nutritious foods 80 percent of the time, you
can eat whatever you want for the remaining 20 percent and not feel guilty. If your diet is consistently
nutritious, an occasional hot dog or milk shake isn't
going to adversely affect you.

**Unfortunately, too many people follow the
20/80 rule.** Those who follow the 20/80 rule have
diets high in calories, fat, saturated fat, cholesterol,
sugar, and sodium, and low in grains, fruits, and vegetables. Knowing their diet is low in nutrients, some
people compensate by adding vitamins, fiber, and an

occasional bean sprout. Though it is wise to consider your nutritional needs carefully, it is not wise to lean on a magic bullet vitamin to rescue an out-of-balance diet. What kind of eater are you? Are you more likely to follow the 80/20 rule, the 20/80 rule, or some other rule?

FAST FOODS

For many people, especially for college students, fast foods have become a way of life. The nutritional value of fast foods, from cheeseburgers to leanburgers, can vary greatly. Breakfast foods, potatoes, whole-wheat breads, salad bars, low-fat meat and milk products, low-calorie foods, and vegetable oils are examples of how fast-food companies have expanded their offerings and made foods more nutritious. Nonetheless, one glance at the menu still finds the majority of fast foods high in calories, fat, saturated fat, cholesterol, sodium, and sugar. Frying foods such as french fries and chicken breasts in oil is one reason for the high level of fat in fast foods.

Many fast-food chains now provide nutritional information for their customers. This information can keep you abreast of your nutrient intake, thereby preventing you from exceeding any maximum levels. Although fast foods can be nutritious, it would be unhealthy and expensive to rely on these foods as your main source of nutrition. **Once again, moderation is the key.**

THE TOP TEN THINGS TO EAT

The results are in! Registered dietitians from the Pittsburgh Dietetic Association got together to answer the question most commonly asked of registered dietitians: What should I eat?

1. **Broccoli:** Like other dark green leafy vegetables, broccoli is loaded with vitamins and minerals and its antioxidant properties may help ward off certain diseases. It is low in sodium, high in fiber, and has few calories—a clear winner!
2. **Breakfast:** For peak performance and lots of energy, eat breakfast. When you skip eating in the morning, your body must draw upon stored glucose (**glycogen**) for its energy. Glycogen may be depleted before lunch, leaving you feeling tired and excessively hungry.
3. **Beans:** A virtual powerhouse of nutrients, beans are high in fiber, protein, iron, folic acid, and complex carbohydrates yet low in fat, sodium, and calories. Beans also help prevent constipation, colon cancer, and heart disease.

4. **Grapefruit:** This food provides a generous supply of vitamin C, which helps with iron absorption, and beta-carotene, an antioxidant. Studies show that people who eat five or more servings of vegetables and fruits a day have half the cancer risk of those who eat only two servings a day.
5. **Skim Milk:** Nonfat and low-fat dairy products are still the best source of calcium, which helps keep bones strong and healthy, and prevents osteoporosis.
6. **Oatmeal:** Patricia Harper, a registered dietitian and coauthor of *Happy Thoughts for a Healthy Life,* advises:

   Eat a little oat bran every day;
   Your cholesterol will go down they say.
   For fiber and regularity, too;
   Wheat bran will do the trick for you.

7. **Round Steak:** Beef can be part of a low-fat diet if you choose lean cuts, trim all visible fat before cooking, and eat small portions (3–4 ounces, cooked). Beef is an excellent source of complete protein, iron, zinc, and vitamin B_{12} nutrients that are sometimes hard to obtain in a vegetarian diet.
8. **Salmon:** Fish is not only low in calories, fat, and sodium but also high in protein and B vitamins. Certain types of fish, such as salmon, tuna, trout, and sardines, have the added advantage of being high in omega-3 fatty acids, an essential nutrient that is thought to be protective against heart disease.
9. **Fig Bars:** Snacking, an All-American pastime, can be part of a healthy diet. Fig bars are low in fat and high in fiber. Other good choices are pretzels, gingersnaps, animal crackers, and graham crackers. Of course, low-fat or fat-free does not mean calorie-free, so be sure to exercise portion control.
10. **Olive Oil:** All fats and oils are not created equal. Using monounsaturated fats such as olive oil and canola oil can help to reduce blood cholesterol level. This, in turn, can reduce heart disease, the number one cause of death in the United States.

FOOD LABELS

Reading food labels is the best way to judge the contributions of individual foods to your daily diet and health goals. Many shoppers compare prices, but few compare labels before selecting foods. In the past, food labels have been confusing and misleading. New regulations by the Food and Drug Administration (FDA) have strict rules governing labels and descriptive terms (see fig. 12.4 and table 12.6).

FIGURE 12.4

Nutrition Facts

New heading signals a new label.

More consistent serving sizes, in both household and metric measures, replace those that used to be set by manufacturers.

New mandatory component helps consumers meet dietary guidelines recommending no more than 30 percent of calories from fat.

Nutrients required on nutrition panel are those most important to the health of today's consumers, most of whom need to worry about getting too much of certain items (fat, for example), rather than too few vitamins or minerals, as in the past.

% Daily Value shows how a food fits into the overall daily diet.

Conversion guide helps consumers learn caloric value of the energy-producing nutrients.

Reference values help consumers learn good diet basics. They can be adjusted, depending on a person's calorie needs.

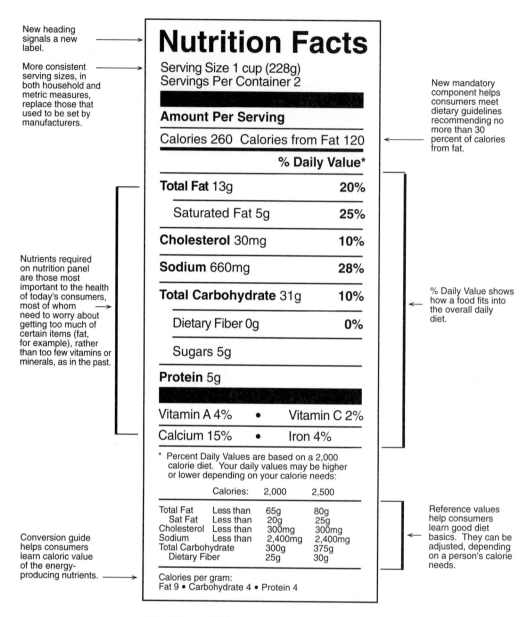

Nutrition Facts

Serving Size 1 cup (228g)
Servings Per Container 2

Amount Per Serving

Calories 260 Calories from Fat 120

% Daily Value*

Total Fat 13g	**20%**
Saturated Fat 5g	**25%**
Cholesterol 30mg	**10%**
Sodium 660mg	**28%**
Total Carbohydrate 31g	**10%**
Dietary Fiber 0g	**0%**
Sugars 5g	
Protein 5g	

Vitamin A 4%	•	Vitamin C 2%	
Calcium 15%	•	Iron 4%	

* Percent Daily Values are based on a 2,000 calorie diet. Your daily values may be higher or lower depending on your calorie needs:

		Calories:	2,000	2,500
Total Fat	Less than		65g	80g
Sat Fat	Less than		20g	25g
Cholesterol	Less than		300mg	300mg
Sodium	Less than		2,400mg	2,400mg
Total Carbohydrate			300g	375g
Dietary Fiber			25g	30g

Calories per gram:
Fat 9 • Carbohydrate 4 • Protein 4

Note: The new labeling rules won't apply to fresh meat, poultry, and fish; fresh fruits and vegetables; and restaurant food. Thus restaurants will, for instance, still be able to use terms like "low-fat" any way they like, though consumer groups are fighting this exemption.

SUMMARY

- Nutrition is defined as the science of food, its use within the body, and its relationship to good health.
- Nutrition involves the study of approximately forty-six essential nutrients, which fall into six major categories: carbohydrates, proteins, fats, vitamins, minerals, and water.
- Proper nutrition is considered an important component for a healthy lifestyle.

- Hunger is the physiological need for food, whereas appetite is the desire to eat. To promote good health, people need to learn to control appetite.
- Food affects all dimensions of wellness.
- A Calorie or kilocalorie is used to indicate the energy value of food.
- Carbohydrates are the ideal fuel source for the body, contributing to about half of the body's energy needs.

TABLE 12.6
New FDA Regulations for Nutrition Labeling

Descriptive Term	Definition
Calorie free	Less than 5 calories per serving
Low calorie	No more than 40 calories per serving and no more than 0.4 calories per gram
Sugar free	Less than 0.5 grams per serving
Sodium/salt free	Less than 5 milligrams per serving
Very low sodium	Less than 35 milligrams per serving
Low sodium	Less than 140 milligrams per serving
Lite/light/lightly	⅓ fewer calories or less fat, salt, sodium, or breading than a similar product
Fat free	Less than 0.5 grams per serving
Low fat	3 grams or less per serving
Low saturated fat	1 gram or less of saturated fat per serving, not more than 15% of total calories
Leaner/lower fat/less fat	At least 25% reduction in fat or an increase in lean content in a suitable comparison
Percent fat free	Based on percent of fat by total weight—refers to portion of the product that is not fat (lean)
Cholesterol free/no cholesterol	Less than 2 milligrams per serving
Low cholesterol	Less than 21 milligrams per 3.5 ounces (100 grams)
Reduced cholesterol	At least 75% less cholesterol per serving than original product
Source of dietary fiber	10 to 19 percent of Daily Reference Values of fiber
High source of dietary fiber	20 percent or more of Daily Reference Values of fiber

- Fiber, a carbohydrate, is associated with many health benefits even though it contains no calories or energy for the body.
- A small amount of fat in the diet is required for good health. Experts recommend no more than 30 percent of daily calories should come from fat.
- The two types of fats are saturated and unsaturated.
- Cholesterol is a waxy, fatlike substance that is essential for life. It is carried in the bloodstream by low-density (bad cholesterol) and high-density (good cholesterol) lipoproteins.
- An increase in the foods containing antioxidants and a decrease in the foods high in saturated fat may lower cholesterol levels.
- Proteins are needed for growth, repair, and maintenance of all body cells.
- Vitamins are organic substances needed by the body in trace amounts. Although most people do not need vitamin supplements, those who do include some vegetarians, pregnant or breast-feeding women, women with excessive menstrual bleeding, strict dieters, and those who do not eat healthfully.
- Folic acid has become increasingly important in the diet to help prevent birth defects and the risk for heart disease and stroke.
- Minerals perform many vital functions in the body, from building strong bones and teeth to forming hemoglobin in the red blood cells.
- Water is often called the "forgotten nutrient," yet is our most important one, since we could not live more than a week without it.
- A new Food Guide Pyramid is now being used to help you choose the correct number of servings from each of the five food groups.
- Newly revised dietary guidelines for Americans include (1) a varied diet, (2) exercise, (3) weight maintenance, and (4) drinking alcohol in moderation.
- The 80/20 rule is another guide for healthy nutrition. This rule states that if you eat a variety of nutritious foods 80 percent of the time, you can eat whatever you want for the remaining 20 percent and not feel guilty.
- Fast foods have become a way of life for many people, especially for college students. The nutritional value of many fast foods has improved greatly, but most are still high in calories, fat, saturated fat, sodium, and sugars.
- Reading food labels is the best way to judge the contributions of individual foods to your daily diet and health goals.

A C T I V I T Y   *12A*

NUTRITION QUESTIONNAIRE

Name _____   *To be submitted:*   Yes   No

Date _____   *If yes, due date* _____

Class _____ Section _____   *Score* _____

PURPOSE

1. To evaluate how well you eat.

2. To determine your strengths and weaknesses in the following seven dietary guidelines for healthy eating.

DIRECTIONS

1. Answer the questions of the Nutrition Questionnaire by placing the appropriate points in the score column.

2. Add up your scores for each guideline and write them in the Results section.

3. Answer the questions in the Results section.

Part A. Eat a Variety of Foods

Do you eat a variety of healthy foods each day? For each question, give yourself 2 points if your answer is *always,* 1 point if your answer is *usually,* and 0 points if your answer is *seldom or never.* Maximum possible points = 10.

Score

1. _____ I eat at least six servings every day from the breads, cereals, rice, and pasta group.

2. _____ I eat at least three servings every day from the vegetable group.

3. _____ I eat at least two servings every day from the fruits group.

4. _____ I have a minimum of two but not more than three servings each day from the milk, yogurt, and cheese group (keep the point if your servings above three are low-fat).

5. _____ I have a minimum of two but not more than three servings each day from the meat, poultry, fish, dry beans, and nuts group.

_____ Total

Part B. Maintain Healthy Weight

Are you maintaining a healthy weight? If you are, give yourself 10 points. If not, give yourself 0 points. Maximum possible points = 10.

1. _____ Are you within your recommended weight range? See table 8.4 on page 105.

_____ Total

Part C. Choose a Diet Low in Fat, Saturated Fat, and Cholesterol

Is your diet low in fat, saturated fat, and cholesterol? Give yourself 1 point for every *yes* answer and 0 points for every *no* answer. Maximum possible points = 10.

1. _____ My milk, yogurt, and cheese selections are mostly nonfat or low in fat (low-fat milk for whole milk, mozzarella cheese for cheddar cheese).

2. _____ I use margarine, butter, cream, or sour cream sparingly or not at all.

3. _____ I keep my servings from the meat, poultry, fish, dry beans, eggs, and nuts group to two moderate servings each day and occasionally have meatless meals.

4. _____ Before cooking and especially before eating, I remove the skin from chicken and visible fat from meat.

5. _____ I eat more fish and chicken than beef, ham, lamb, or pork.

6. _____ In preparing or ordering beef, fish, or chicken, I choose grilling, broiling, and baking over frying.

7. _____ I choose low-fat yogurt, sherbet, or ice milk over ice cream.

8. _____ I use as little salad dressing as possible for my salads.

9. _____ When eating fast foods, I choose low-fat products (salad and fruit bar, baked potato, water) over high-fat products (cheeseburgers, french fries, shakes).

10. _____ I limit high-fat snacks and deserts (cookies, cakes, ice cream).

_____ Total

Part D. Choose a Diet with Plenty of Vegetables, Fruits, and Grain Products

Is your diet loaded with vegetables, fruits, and grains? For every *yes* answer, give yourself 1 point. For every *no* answer, give yourself 0 points. Maximum possible points = 10.

1. _____ I like the taste of vegetables and enjoy eating them daily.

2. _____ I like the taste of fruits and enjoy eating them daily.

3. _____ I would prefer choosing a vegetable or fruit snack over any other snack.

4. _____ If the option were available, I would choose fruit dessert over any other dessert.

5. _____ If I realize during the evening that I have not consumed the recommended daily number of vegetable (three) and fruit (two) servings, I will strive to correct the deficiency that night or the next day.

6. _____ If the option were available, I would choose a wheat or bran cereal over a presweetened cereal.

7. _____ If the option were available, I would choose whole-wheat bread over white bread.

8. _____ I eat products from a variety of grains, such as wheat, rice, and oats, as well as pasta.

9. _____ I limit high-fat grains in my diet (croissants, cakes, cookies).

10. _____ I strive to eat a minimum of six servings each day from bread, cereal, rice, and pasta products.

_____ Total

Part E. Use Sugars Only in Moderation

What size (small, medium, large, or humongous) is your sweet tooth? For every *yes* answer, give yourself 1 point. For every *no* answer, give yourself 0 points. Maximum possible points = 5.

1. _____ I limit sugar intake whenever possible.

2. _____ I eat candy or chocolate seldomly or not at all.

3. _____ I would prefer cereal, tea, and coffee with no sugar or sweeteners added. (Keep the point if you don't eat cereal or drink tea or coffee.)

4. _____ I drink more water and milk than sweetened liquids such as Kool-Aid and soft drinks.

5. _____ I choose snacks that are either no-sugar, low-sugar, or natural sugar (vegetables, fruits) over high-sugar snacks and desserts (cookies, cakes).

_____ Total

Part F. Use Salt and Sodium Only in Moderation

What mountain (small, medium, or high) of salt are you on? If your answer is *always,* give yourself 2 points. If your answer is *usually,* give yourself 1 point, and if your answer is *seldom or never* give yourself 0 points. Maximum possible points = 4.

1. _____ I choose foods lightly salted or not salted at all.

2. _____ I add little or no salt while cooking foods or when eating them.

_____ Total

Part G. If You Drink Alcoholic Beverages, Do So in Moderation

If you do drink alcohol, do you drink in moderation? For every *yes* answer, give yourself 5 points. If your answer is *no,* give yourself 0 points. Maximum possible points = 10.

1. _____ I do not drink more than two alcoholic beverages in a day. One drink is 5 oz. of wine, 10 oz. of wine cooler, 12 oz. of beer, or 1 oz. of hard liquor (whiskey, gin, rum, vodka).

2. _____ I rarely or never skip entire meals or major portions of meals because my stomach is full from drinking alcoholic beverages.

_____ Total

RESULTS

After totaling your scores for each part, write them on the blanks below.

Part A. _____

Part B. _____

Part C. _____

Part D. _____

Part E. _____

Part F. _____

Part G. _____

Total _____ (out of 59)

Rating _____

Ratings

55–59   Superior food selection.

48–54   Healthy food selection.

40–47   Okay, but room for improvement.

30–39   Below average. Consider eating for your health and not just for your taste buds.

Below 30   Help! Make an appointment with your instructor, physician, or a dietitian for immediate dietary counseling.

1. Do you feel your rating accurately reflects your nutritional health?   Yes   No   Explain.

2. What dietary guidelines were you strong in?

3. What dietary guidelines, if any, were you weak in?

4. What did you learn from this questionnaire? Will you apply this information to your daily food selections?   Yes   No

ACTIVITY   *12B*

NUTRITION PROJECT

Name _____   **To be submitted: Yes   No**

Date _____   **If yes, due date** _____

Class _____   **Section** _____   **Score** _____

PURPOSE
1. To monitor your food patterns.
2. To determine if you are following the recommended daily servings from the five food groups.

DIRECTIONS
1. Using the form in this activity, monitor your food patterns by recording all food and drink (including water) for the number of days (three to seven) that your instructor has planned.
2. Try not to alter your normal eating patterns during the project. Once the project is over, you're welcome to make changes.
3. In the time column, write down when you consume the food and/or drink.
4. In the Food/Amount/Cal. column, list the food or drink and the amount (estimate if you don't know) you consume (e.g., 3/4 cup cereal, 2 bread slices, 1 medium orange, 1 glass of water). Check with a calorie guide and record the number of calories in each food and drink.
5. Next, identify the food group (grains, vegetables, fruits, dairy, meat group) or food category (fats, oils, sweets) in which each food and drink belongs. Water is not in any food group. Include the number of servings (refer to the Food Guide Pyramid on page 150).
6. In the healthy column, write either Yes (that apple was healthy) or No (that candy bar was not healthy) for each item.
7. Record where you were (cafeteria) and what you were doing (sitting with friends) for each meal or snack.
8. In the next column, write down the mood you were in (happy, sad, lonely, stressed, etc.) for each meal or snack.
9. For the last column, identify your level of hunger before eating by using the following codes:
   1. Very Full
   2. Somewhat Full
   3. Not Full, Not Hungry
   4. Just Now Feeling Hungry
   5. Feelings of Hunger for One or More Hours
10. Answer questions in Results section.

Date _____

Time	Food/Amount/Cal.	Food Group/ # of Servings	Healthy	Where/Doing What?	Mood	Hunger (0–5)

RESULTS

1. Did you notice any patterns related to time and when you snacked?   Yes   No   Explain.

2. For the food group/category column, were you able to satisfy the recommended adult servings for the five food groups?
   Yes   No   If you were deficient, which food groups(s) need additional servings?

3. In your health column, were the majority of foods/drinks you consumed healthy or unhealthy? Estimate your ratio of nutritious foods/drinks to unhealthy foods/drinks (recommended 80/20). What foods could you reduce in your diet and what foods could you add to improve your health?

   Ratio: _____

   Foods to Reduce   Foods to Add
   1. _____   1. _____
   2. _____   2. _____
   3. _____   3. _____
   4. _____   4. _____

4. What did you learn from this project?

CHAPTER 13

STRATEGIES FOR LIFETIME WEIGHT AND FAT CONTROL

Desire + knowledge + skills = your formula for success for lifetime weight and fat control!

LEARNING OBJECTIVES

- Identify the trends with weight and fat gain.

- Examine why dieting by itself does not work.

- Identify and briefly describe the five key strategies for lifetime weight and fat control.

- Define compulsive overeating and learn how to recognize the early warning signs.

- Describe briefly the common eating disorders.

LIFESTYLE QUESTIONS

- Are you satisfied with your present level of body weight?

- Are you satisfied with your present level of body fat?

- Have you ever lost weight by dieting, then stopped the diet and gained the weight back and then some?

- Are you on a diet now?

- Have you ever used exercise as a method to lose weight, then stopped exercising and gained the weight back?

- Would you like to gain weight but find it difficult to do so?

- Generally, do you tend to overeat, undereat, or eat just the right amount of food?

- Do you know someone who is anorexic or bulimic?

INTRODUCTION

Americans spend 33 billion dollars a year on diet books, diet drinks, diet meals, and weight loss programs, according to a new study by the Institute of Medicine. In spite of spending all this money, Americans are being swallowed up in an epidemic of obesity, getting fatter and fatter. In fact, overweight Americans aged 20 to 74 increased from 1 in 4 to 1 in 3 from the end of 1980 to the end of 1990. The study also found that although more than 44 million Americans are trying to lose weight, the majority can't keep it off for more than two years. At the other extreme, the incidence of anorexia and bulimia is also on the rise. These facts demonstrate the complexity of food intake and Americans' preoccupation with their bodies.

THE PROBLEMS WITH DIETING BY ITSELF

Study after study demonstrates that dieting alone does not work for the majority of participants. This is especially true if it is a very-low-calorie diet. The multibillion-dollar diet industry wants you to believe that to lose weight and fat, you just need to follow their special diets. Most diets, however, not only fail to deliver on their guarantees, they can also lead to serious health problems such as low blood pressure, heart disease, and sudden death.

Dieting alone slows the rate of fat loss and may predispose one to a rapid weight gain. The body interprets dietary restrictions as famine and responds in a defensive manner by slowing its metabolic rate and

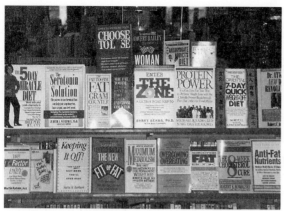

There are numerous diet books on the market—"Let the Buyer Beware."

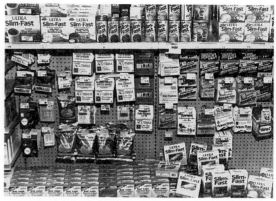

Liquid diets and diet aids may work temporarily but are not a permanent solution.

enhancing its ability to store excess calories as fat. Dieting alone can also tend to use up muscle tissue, which is considered the body's fat burner. Any loss of muscle mass will lower the body's capacity to burn calories and decrease the chances of losing weight.

Analyze a diet carefully before following it. If you come across a diet that promises you the cake, icing, and candles too, evaluate it using the following questions. Stay away from any special diets unless you get all yes responses.

1. Does it encourage a weight loss of no more than one to two pounds a week?
2. Does it encourage physical activity?
3. Does it contain a selection of nutritious foods?
4. Does it emphasize medium-sized portions?
5. Does it use foods that are easy to locate and prepare?
6. Does it give you enough variety?
7. Can you follow it wherever you eat—at home, work, restaurants, or social events?
8. Is the cost reasonable?
9. Can you live on this diet *for the rest of your life?*

Liquid Diets and Diet Aids

Liquid diet aids can be unhealthy and seldom work in the long run. They supply between 420 and 840 calories a day, which can lead to a rapid weight loss. These special diets do provide enough protein to preserve muscle tissue. However, once the dieter stops the program and returns to normal eating patterns, the weight usually returns.

Liquid diets are usually reserved for those who are at least 20 percent over their ideal weight and should only be administered by physicians. Weekly screenings for vital body functions are necessary to determine how the body is responding without solid food. Complications of these low-calorie diets include dry skin, hair loss, constipation, gum disease, sensitivity to cold, and mood swings.

Diet aids—which include pills such as "fen-phen" (a combination of two diet pills), the newest diet pill, Redux, and diet gum—low- or no-calorie soft drinks, and low-calorie foods may work temporarily, but they are not a permanent solution.

STRATEGIES FOR LIFETIME WEIGHT AND FAT CONTROL

The key to permanent fat control is a new lifestyle approach that is flexible, accepting, and family-based. It discourages calorie counting and food-focused programs that encourage dieting. The act of losing weight and fat poses certain health risks such as cardiovascular disease, high blood pressure, diabetes, and sleep apnea. Due to these potential dangers, experts strongly recommend a consultation with a physician before and during any program. This new lifestyle includes five important strategies: (1) Get Psyched! (2) Get Nutritionally Aware! (3) Change Unhealthy Behaviors! (4) Get Physically Active! and (5) Get Support!

Get Psyched!

Motivation is the drive or desire to begin or continue a behavior. It is the first step in a lifetime weight and fat control program. Your success will be determined, in large part, by your level of motivation. The more motivated you are, the better your chance of success. If you're self-motivated, you strive to reach your goals for internal rewards. Experts in goal attainment believe internal rewards such as self-esteem and self-confidence are more powerful than external rewards such as money and gifts. Whether you use one type of reward over the other, or combine both, the key is to use whatever works for you. See table 13.1 for tips on motivation.

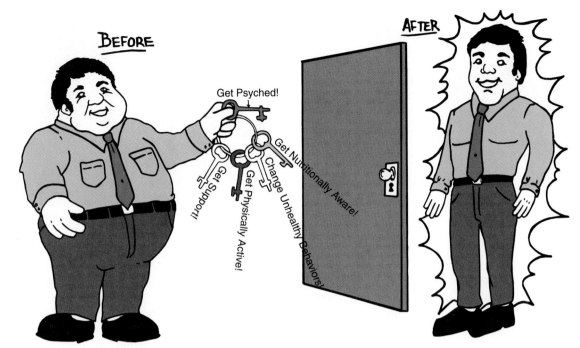

Keys to lifetime fat control.

TABLE 13.1

Motivational Tips for Weight and Fat Control

1. Think positively. Know you can and will do it. Think about the new you—feeling, looking, and functioning better, with improved health and a better quality of life.

2. Use rewards. When you reach your goals, give yourself compliments ("I did it!" and "Way to go!"). Buy something nice for yourself, too.

3. Write down at least five reasons why you want to lose weight and fat and read them daily.

4. Set realistic goals in terms of how much you expect to lose and by when you expect to lose it. Experts recommend losing no more than 1 to 2 pounds a week.

5. Visualize yourself with your new body six months from now and one year from now.

6. Write out a contract. This will raise your level of commitment.

Get Nutritionally Aware!

Since eating is one of life's pleasures, it is important to have a basic understanding of nutrition for making sensible, well-balanced food selections. The same guidelines for good nutrition can be applied to guidelines for lifetime fat control. These include eating low amounts of fat, saturated fat, cholesterol, sugar, and salt; eating high amounts of complex carbohydrates, vegetables, fruits, and fiber; and establishing healthy food relationships.

Reducing dietary fat will eliminate an enormous amount of extra calories and lead to better health. Every gram of fat you consume is equal to nine Calories. This is more than double the four Calories each in one gram of carbohydrates and in one gram of protein. Plus, the more fat in your diet, the higher your risk of heart disease and some cancers. This is true even if you're not overfat.

Follow the Food Guide Pyramid and use smaller portions. A well-balanced diet is your source of dynamic energy. When losing weight and fat, your body still needs the nutrients and Calories necessary for optimal functioning. The Food Guide Pyramid (see figure 12.3 in chapter 12) will serve as a program to follow in choosing nutritious foods. Also, smaller portions of the daily recommended servings are helpful to reduce the number of Calories.

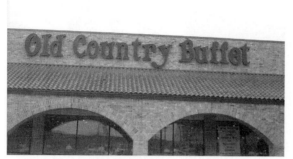

Eating at buffets is hazardous to your waistline.

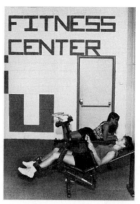

Weight training

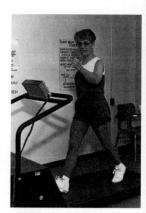

Treadmill walking

Change Unhealthy Behaviors!

Eating behavior is influenced by physical, emotional, and social factors. Why do you eat? Is it only because you are hungry? When do you eat? Is it only at mealtimes? Or when you are happy? Sad? Bored? With others? By yourself? In front of the television? While you read? When you drink? When you're upset? Angry? When you celebrate? When you are depressed? Your answers may indicate that your eating patterns are dictated by factors other than hunger. Knowing why you eat and what provokes you to eat will help you improve your eating habits.

Modifying or changing your behaviors (behavior modification) is the cornerstone for a program of lifetime weight and fat control. It is built on the idea that all behaviors are learned responses from environmental cues or previous experiences. As you learn to change unhealthy habits (e.g., going back for seconds), eating becomes a more conscious act and healthy habits are adopted (e.g., eating more slowly). Table 13.2 provides examples of strategies for modifying behavior. Which ones could you employ to become a healthier eater?

Get Physically Active!

Recent evidence indicates that obesity is more dependent on inactivity than on overeating. Although we eat fewer calories than Americans did in the early 1900s, we are much fatter. Why? Because activity levels have declined significantly. Elevators, riding lawn mowers, power tools, remote controls, and mobile phones are just a few examples of how technology has stripped us from using more calories. Due to the sedentary American way of life, it is vital to engage in voluntary physical activity as a strategy for fat loss.

The most significant factor in achieving lifetime weight and fat control is regular, moderate exercise and strength training. The American College of Sports Medicine recommends two forms of exercise for fat loss: aerobic exercise and strength-training activities like weight lifting. Aerobic activities such as walking, jogging, bicycling, swimming, dancing, and cross-country skiing are excellent calorie-burning exercises because they are performed continuously for long periods of time. Table 13.3 shows the calories expended per hour in various physical activities. Strength training or resistance exercise (weights, sit-ups, push-ups) will help increase muscle tissue, thereby increasing metabolism and using more calories. Besides using more calories, strength exercises will also shrink the size of fat cells.

To complement the fat-loss effects of aerobic exercise and strength training, become more active in your leisure time. To give a boost to your fat control program, you can watch less television, drive less, walk more, use stairs, plant a garden, play with the dog, and participate in active sports. The contributions of exercise to weight and fat loss are found in table 13.4.

To promote long-term adherence and reduce weight and body fat, follow the FITT exercise formula (see chapter 4). Many motivated participants, eager to lose weight and fat, start out their exercise programs incorrectly by doing too much too soon. The obvious result: another dropout statistic. Follow the exercise guidelines found in table 8.2 for a safe and effective way to reduce body fat.

At the beginning of an exercise program, a loss of inches and body fat will occur, but not necessarily weight. During the first six to eight weeks of your exercise program, you may not lose any weight. Since muscle weighs more than fat, you may actually experience a slight increase in body weight during this time period. However, because the weight gained is muscle and the weight lost is fat, you will be healthier and should experience a decrease in body circumference measurements. Beginning exercisers will often lose inches and have their clothes fit better while remaining at the same weight.

TABLE 13.2

Behavioral Strategies for Weight and Fat Control

1. Keep a food diary to determine eating patterns.

2. Satisfy your hunger with vegetables, fruits, and grains before eating fatty foods and sweets.

3. Slow down so that your appetite controls how much you eat. Be "in touch" with your fullness level.

4. Eat only when you are physically hungry.

5. Plan your meals in advance.

6. Concentrate only on eating. If you watch television or read while you eat, you may tend to eat more.

7. Reinforce your new healthy habits by giving yourself a pat on the back and other nice rewards.

8. Learn to relax when eating. Instead of eating when you're upset, angry, or under stress, go for a walk or listen to a relaxation tape.

9. Substitute other activities for snacking. Take a walk, read, call a friend, write a term paper, fly a kite, clean your room, etc.

10. Plan for holidays and other special occasions. If you know you're going to overeat, exercise twice that day, or lower calorie intake and exercise more the day before or the day after.

11. Use smaller plates and chew food slowly.

12. Only eat at the table. *Never* eat standing up.

13. Use self-discipline. Keep problem food (chips, sweets) out of sight and out of mind.

14. Keep nutritious food in sight and in mind.

15. Think of food as fuel for the body, instead of simply pleasure for the taste buds.

16. If you lapse (overeating, junking out) for a meal or a day, simply return to your program—think of it as a learning experience.

17. Eat breakfast. It appears that breakfast prevents hunger and subsequent overeating, reduces the amount of overall fat eaten, and helps control impulsive snacking.

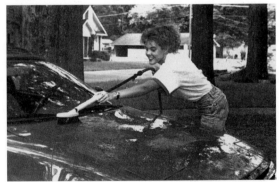
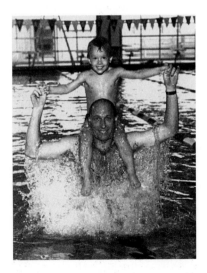

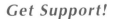
Being active throughout the day can help with fat control: (1) Washing your car (2) Having fun with children

Get Support!

Support from family, friends, and groups is an important piece of the weight/fat-control puzzle. No question about it—losing weight and fat is no easy task. The more ammunition you have in your arsenal, the better your chances of success. To improve your odds, enlist the support of family, friends, roommates, and groups. Maybe you can enlist a friend or family member who also wants to lose unwanted pounds and inches. Although the cheering of others can be crucial to your success, the most important support must come from you. With your personal commitment in place, your mission can be accomplished. See table 13.5 for strategies to create a supportive environment.

TABLE 13.3

Calories Expended per Hour in Various Activities (Performed at a Recreational Level)*

Intensity Level⁺		Calories Used per Hour				
	Activity	*100 lbs.*	*120 lbs.*	*150 lbs.*	*180 lbs.*	*200 lbs.*
Low	Pool; billiards	97	110	130	150	163
	Sailing (pleasure)	135	153	180	207	225
	Bowling	155	176	208	240	261
	Bicycling (normal speed)	157	178	210	242	263
	Social dance	174	222	264	318	348
	Archery	180	204	240	276	300
	Horseback riding	180	204	240	276	300
	Table tennis	180	204	240	276	300
	Golf (walking)	187	212	250	288	313
	Walking	204	258	318	372	426
	Baseball	210	238	280	322	350
	Softball (fast)	210	238	280	322	350
	Softball (slow)	217	246	290	334	363
	Basketball (half-court)	225	255	300	345	375
	Fencing	225	255	300	345	375
	Football	225	255	300	345	375
	Hiking	225	255	300	345	375
	Fitness calisthenics	232	263	310	357	388
	Gymnastics	232	263	310	357	388
	Judo/karate	232	263	310	357	388
	Modern dance	240	300	360	432	480
	Ballet dance	240	300	360	432	480
Moderate	Swimming (slow laps)	240	272	320	368	400
	Circuit training	247	280	330	380	413
	Badminton	255	289	340	391	425
	Ice skating	262	297	350	403	438
	Roller skating	262	297	350	403	438
	Volleyball	262	297	350	403	438
	Canoeing (4 mph)	276	344	414	504	558
	Waterskiing	306	390	468	564	636
	Backpacking (40 lb. pack)	307	348	410	472	513
	Tennis	315	357	420	483	525
	Exercise dance	315	357	420	483	525
	Weight training	352	399	470	541	558
High	Soccer	405	459	540	621	775
	Surfing	416	467	550	633	684
	Swimming (fast laps)	420	530	630	768	846
	Skiing downhill	450	510	600	690	750
	Handball	450	510	600	690	750
	Mountain climbing	450	510	600	690	750
	Racquetball	450	510	600	690	750
	Paddleball	450	510	600	690	750
	Interval training	487	552	650	748	833
	Jogging (5½ mph)	487	552	650	748	833
	Cross-country skiing	525	595	700	805	875
	Rope jumping (continuous)	525	595	700	805	875
	Rowing, crew	615	697	820	943	1025
	Running (10 mph)	625	765	900	1035	1125

*Note: Locate your weight to determine the calories used per hour in each of the activities shown in the table based on recreational involvement. Based on research completed at the Human Performance Laboratory, Brigham Young University.

⁺Note: There is no clear line of separation. Most activities are not inherently low or high intensity (except in activities like pool and bowling). How the activities are played is the deciding factor. The amount of calories burned in any activity depends on: (1) skill level of participants and (2) movement intensity.

TABLE 13.4
Contributions of Exercise to Weight and Fat Loss

1. **Uses Calories.** Aerobic exercise can be done at a comfortable pace for 30 to 60 minutes. With each minute of activity, you're using up more calories than you would be at rest.

2. **Increase Basal Metabolic Rate.** If you do plan to diet, exercise can help keep your BMR up when your body wants to slow it down. After finishing a workout, your metabolic rate is increased for several hours, continuing to use calories at a faster pace.

3. **Shrinks Fat Cells.** Exercise can reduce the size of the fat cells. Based on current scientific evidence, it does not appear that you can reduce the number of fat cells. However, you can shrink their size and lower your percent body fat.

4. **Prevents Loss of Muscle.** Resistant exercises such as weight training accelerate the rate of muscle buildup.

TABLE 13.5
Strategies for a Supportive Environment

1. Recruit at least one friend or family member who will stand by you at all times. Make out a contract and have this person sign it.

2. Announce your weight and fat control plans to as many people as possible. You will be more committed and will not want to let them down.

3. Make a game out of it. For every centimeter (ounce, inch, pound) you lose, you receive a dollar from your support team. Of course, if gains occur, you pay.

4. Stay in contact with those supporting you. Share your successes. Lean on them during difficult times.

5. Plan a celebration event for your success with your support team. Then carry it out after you reach your goals.

6. Join a support group.

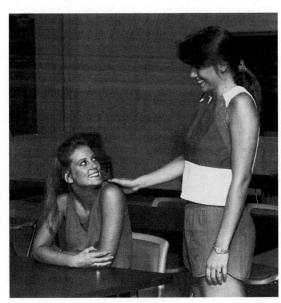

Receiving support from others is a powerful strategy for weight and fat management.

TOO GOOD TO BE TRUE?

Recent evidence has found that a natural fat-busting protein named leptin slimmed down overweight mice. This exciting finding, of course, has far-reaching implications for overweight people. However, new research indicates that very obese people already have high levels of leptin in their bodies, so injecting more may not help at all. On the other side, the very obese may just need more of this fat-busting protein injected to control their weight. More investigation is needed to determine whether leptin can work in overweight humans.

RELAPSES

Although relapses are common among participants engaging in behavior change, they can serve as learning experiences to build upon for future success. When attempting a health change, it's almost inevitable for most people to relapse and revert back to old, unhealthy habits. The three most common reasons for relapse are: (1) stress-related factors (major life changes, depression, job and school changes, and illness); (2) social factors (travel, eating out, entertaining); and (3) self-enticing behaviors, such as putting yourself in positions to determine how much you can get away with (e.g., "one bite of ice cream won't hurt me," leading to "I'll just have one scoop," and finally, "I haven't done so well, I might as well eat the whole gallon").

Falling back to old behaviors is part of being human. If you slip back, know why and learn from the experience. Feeling guilt or anger toward yourself for not sticking with it may hinder your efforts. Just simply pick yourself up and get back on track. If you have the will, and blend it with perseverance, you will be successful with your weight and fat reduction goals. The rewards await you.

MAINTAINING DESIRABLE WEIGHT AND FAT

Once you have arrived at your desirable weight and body fat level, you are only halfway there. The challenge now is to achieve weight and fat maintenance for the rest of your life. The solution is a healthy, active lifestyle, including the five keys to lifetime weight and fat control.

GAINING WEIGHT

Those who need to gain weight can benefit from a change in their eating and exercise patterns. Most people who desire to gain weight want to gain lean body tissue (muscle), not fat tissue. Only those who have body fat percentages below 10 percent for women and 5 percent for men will want to gain additional fat. For weight gain, consume more calories from complex carbohydrates such as pasta, rice, bread, potatoes, and cereals. In addition to a high-carbohydrate diet, regular exercise (including strength training) can add weight by increasing muscle.

COMPULSIVE OVEREATING

As with other addictive behaviors (gambling, smoking), compulsive overeating is characterized by a lack of control. Evidence suggests that food addicts may process foods differently than do normal eaters. Once they begin to eat, they lack control over this act and find it difficult to stop. Compulsive eaters often choose sweets and foods high in sugar, which boosts the level of serotonin, a brain chemical that affects mood and emotion. As addiction sets in, they become preoccupied with eating these foods and use them to change their mood or avoid their problems.

Food addicts will continue to overeat in spite of weight gain. By cutting back or eliminating these foods, they experience common withdrawal symptoms such as depression, irritability, fatigue, insomnia, nausea, headaches, and severe mood swings (see table 13.6 for early warning signs of compulsive overeating).

Total recovery is difficult, because compulsive eaters cannot give up their "substance" entirely. Learning new eating patterns and dealing with underlying emotional problems are the steps to recovery for compulsive overeaters. Doctors, nutritionists, therapists, and support groups like Overeaters Anonymous are helpful in overcoming this addiction. Therapy includes avoiding foods that set off cravings, learning to eat to live, rather than living to eat, and by using food as fuel for the body.

TABLE 13.6
Early Warning Signs of Compulsive Overeating

1. Turning to food when depressed or lonely, when feeling rejected, or as a reward.
2. A history of failed diets.
3. Preoccupied with food throughout the day.
4. Eating quickly and without pleasure.
5. Frequent talking about food, or refusing to talk about food.
6. Fear of not being able to stop eating.
7. Continuing to eat when stomach is full.
8. Experiencing stress when eating.
9. Body weight is 10 percent or more above ideal weight.

EATING DISORDERS

The current emphasis on physical attractiveness in our society has increased the frequency of eating disorders. Thin is in and fat is out. Fear of fatness in our society has resulted in an obsession with thinness. The excessive desire to be thin has led to an increase in the eating disorders of anorexia nervosa, bulimia, and bulimarexia.

All eating disorders are considered serious health problems. Each condition involves the severe restriction of food intake and/or regurgitation of food. Eating disorders are most commonly found among achievement-oriented female adolescents and young women. For males, there is a higher than normal incidence among models, dancers, wrestlers, and long-distance runners.

Anorexia Nervosa

Of the eating disorders, anorexia nervosa is the most serious. Anorectics strive to attain excessive thinness by severely restricting Calories, exercising compulsively, or using laxatives to prevent food digestion. Although they already possess a low percent body fat, they falsely perceive their bodies as being fat (see table 13.7 for common symptoms of anorexia). It is imperative that individuals displaying any of these symptoms seek immediate medical and psychological help, as this condition can lead to serious health problems and, eventually, to death.

Bulimia

The most common of all eating disorders, bulimia is characterized by a compulsive need to consume large quantities of food (bingeing), followed by purging through vomiting, laxatives, or fasting.

TABLE 13.7

Common Symptoms of Anorexia Nervosa

1. A distorted body image.

2. An intense fear of gaining weight or becoming fat.

3. At least a 25 percent loss of original body weight without a known illness accounting for the loss.

4. A refusal to maintain normal body weight.

5. Unusual eating rituals or patterns.

6. In women, absence of at least three menstrual cycles.

TABLE 13.8

Common Symptoms of Bulimia

1. Repeated episodes of binge eating.

2. Lack of control over eating behavior during binges.

3. Regularly engages in self-induced vomiting, fasting, use of laxatives or diuretics, and exercises vigorously to prevent weight gain.

4. An average of two binge eating episodes a week for at least three months.

5. Preoccupation with body shape and weight.

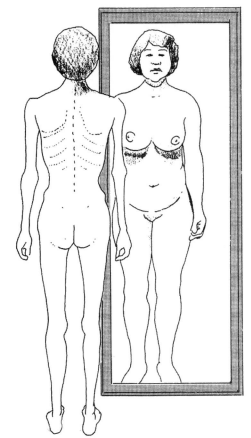

Anorexics have a distorted self-image. Even when they have become dangerously thin, they see themselves as too fat.

Bulimics can appear healthy looking and well-adjusted, often enjoying food and socializing around it. However, their feelings of self-worth and self-confidence are low, smothered by eating binges. Bulimia can begin as voluntary dieting behavior, later becoming compulsive, uncontrollable, and pathological due to emotional repression.

As a result of stressful life events or a compulsion to eat, bulimics can consume thousands of Calories at one sitting, often lasting for an hour or longer. After bingeing, feelings of guilt, shame, and depression emerge, along with the intense fear of weight gain. To reduce anxieties and fears, the bulimic purges. Then the cycle repeats itself. Table 13.8 provides common symptoms of bulimia.

Usually aware of their actions, bulimics have a fear of not being able to stop the binge-and-purge cycle. Unlike anorectics, bulimics realize that their behavior is abnormal and feel ashamed. Because bulimics fear rejection from others, they carry out their habit in secrecy, often during unusual hours of the day. Nevertheless, bulimia can be treated successfully by acknowledging the behavior as self-defeating and as not the solution to life's problems. Professional intervention is strongly recommended. Psychotherapists are helpful in understanding the under-

lying causes and can help reshape the bulimic's feelings of self-worth and self-confidence.

Bulimarexia

Combined symptoms of anorexia nervosa and bulimia is called bulimarexia. Between 40 and 50 percent of people with anorexia exhibit bulimic behavior. Binge eating, purging, and self-starvation with severe weight loss characterize bulimarexia. Immediate professional intervention is crucial to prevent further health problems and for a return to a healthy lifestyle.

SUMMARY

- Obesity is at epidemic proportions in America. Americans are getting fatter and fatter.
- Dieting without exercising does not usually work and can be harmful.
- The five key strategies for lifetime weight and fat control are: (1) Get Psyched! (2) Get Nutritionally Aware! (3) Change Unhealthy Behaviors! (4) Get Physically Active! and (5) Get Support!

- Relapses are common anytime people attempt to change their behavior. The key is to persevere and get back on track!
- Once you have reached your desired weight and body fat level, the challenge is to stay there. Physical activity and a regular fitness program are two important keys.
- To gain weight, include more complex carbohydrates in your diet and more exercise, including strength training.

- Compulsive overeating is an addiction in which the individual lacks self-control over the act of eating.
- The excessive desire to be thin has led to an increase in the eating disorders of anorexia nervosa, bulimia, and bulimarexia. Each one is a serious health condition that needs professional intervention.

A C T I V I T Y   *13A*

DESIGNING YOUR PERSONAL WEIGHT AND FAT CONTROL PROGRAM

Name _____   **To be submitted: Yes   No**

Date _____   **If yes, due date** _____

Class _____   **Section** _____   **Score** _____

PURPOSE

To design your own weight and fat control program. Whether you plan to lose, maintain, or gain weight and fat, this contract will be helpful in reaching your goals. Refer back to chapter 13 to answer the following questions.

DIRECTIONS

1. Fill out the weight and fat control contract, referring to the information in chapter 13.

2. Stick with your program a minimum of three weeks.

3. Once the designated time period for the contract has been completed, answer the questions in the Results section.

4. While this lab only lasts three weeks, maintaining desirable weight and fat control is a lifetime program.

WEIGHT AND FAT CONTROL CONTRACT

I, _____, commit myself to a weight and fat management program for a minimum of three weeks
        (your name)

beginning _____ and ending _____. I plan to _____ _____ or maintain my current weight and level of fat.
     (date)   (date)   (lose/gain   pounds/inches)

1. **Get Psyched!**
   Which motivational tips do you plan to use? (Refer to page 162).

   1. _____

   2. _____

   3. _____

   4. _____

   5. _____

2. **Get Nutritionally Aware!**
   Which nutritional strategies do you plan to use to eat better? (Refer to page 163).

   1. _____

   2. _____

   3. _____

   4. _____

   5. _____

3. **Change Unhealthy Behaviors!**
   Which behavior modification strategies do you plan to eliminate and/or adopt to develop better eating patterns? (Refer to page 164).

   1. _____

   2. _____

   3. _____

   4. _____

   5. _____

4. **Get Physically Active!**
   Check those exercise guidelines you plan to follow:

   Frequency: 5 to 7 days a week   _____

   Intensity: Elevate the heart rate   _____

   Time: 30 to 60 minutes   _____

   Type: Aerobic   _____

   Start Slowly: Gradual buildup   _____

   Weight Training: Light weights, many reps   _____

   Which form(s) of exercise (walking, swimming, bicycling, dancing, jogging, or other) are you most likely to stay with?

   _____

   _____

   _____

5. **Get Support!**
   Have your support team (family, friends, and others) write their names on the lines below, signifying their support for your program.

   _____

   _____

   _____

   _____

   _____

   _____

   _____

RESULTS

1. How did you do with your program?

2. Do you plan to stay with this program?   Yes   No   If so, for how long?

3. Is writing out a contract for a desired health change beneficial to you?   Yes   No   Explain.

ACTIVITY 13B

ARE YOU AT RISK FOR EATING DISORDERS?

Name _____ To be submitted: Yes No

Date _____ If yes, due date _____

Class _____ Section _____ Score _____

PURPOSE
To determine if you are at risk for the eating disorders of anorexia and/or bulimia.

DIRECTIONS
1. Read the following statements in the questionnaire and check all those that apply to you.

EATING DISORDER QUESTIONNAIRE

Anorexia

_____ 1. I see myself as being fat even though I know I'm not.
_____ 2. I have an intense fear of gaining weight or becoming fat.
_____ 3. I have lost 25 percent or more of my original body weight without a known illness accounting for the loss.
_____ 4. I simply refuse to maintain my normal body weight even though I am significantly underweight.
_____ 5. I have unusual rituals or patterns to lose weight including but not limited to excessive exercising and/or using diuretics to lose weight.
_____ 6. For women: I have missed my menstrual cycle for three consecutive months.
_____ 7. I am often self-critical and a perfectionist.
_____ 8. Occasionally, I have binges followed by severe fasts.
_____ 9. I have a fear of independence, intimacy, and adult responsibility.
_____ 10. I have severe sleep disturbances.
_____ 11. I am in pain.

Bulimia

_____ 12. I have repeated episodes of binge eating.
_____ 13. I have lack of control over my eating behavior during binges.
_____ 14. I regularly engage in self-induced vomiting, use of laxatives or diuretics, and/or exercise vigorously to prevent weight gain.
_____ 15. I have a preoccupation with my body shape and weight.
_____ 16. I have low self-esteem.
_____ 17. I have digestive discomfort, indigestion, cramps, pain, bloating, gas, and/or constipation.
_____ 18. I have a strong desire for approval of others.
_____ 19. I am a perfectionist, self-critical, and have excessively high standards.

SCORING
Every statement checked may indicate a likelihood of developing an eating disorder. The more statements checked, the more chance there is. Your college or university will likely have qualified personnel in the student health center or counseling center to advise you.

RESULTS
1. Do you feel you have problems with your eating, dieting, and body? Yes No Explain.

2. Do you know someone whom you perceive as having a problem with an eating disorder? Yes No If yes, is this person seeking any help?

CHAPTER

STRATEGIES TO MANAGE STRESS

A balanced state of stress—not too much and not too little—can lead to health, happiness, and success!

LEARNING OBJECTIVES

- Define stress and stressors.
- Describe the symptoms and health problems that are linked to distress.
- Distinguish among the different types of stress.
- Define and identify different types of stressors.

- Examine the three stages of the stress response.
- Identify the common sources of stressors.
- Explain why daily hassles can lead to more health problems than major life events.

- Discuss the relationship between stress and the different types of personality traits.
- Adopt several healthy coping strategies and relaxation techniques to daily living.

LIFESTYLE QUESTIONS

- Generally speaking, do you manage the stress in your life well?
- Are you easily stressed out?
- Have you ever suffered from a stress-related condition such as ulcers and headaches?

- What are the major and minor stressors in your life today?
- What stress management techniques do you use to manage the stress in your life (i.e., exercise, meditation)?

INTRODUCTION

Stress has become a familiar topic in today's society. What is it? What causes it? How do you know that you have too much? Too little? Or just the right amount? What health problems are linked to it? How do you manage it? And, most important, are you in control of it?

To be alive means to experience stress. It is a normal and natural part of life. Each day you are exposed to and deal with many situations, events, people, and opportunities that can lead to stress. How effectively you cope with daily stress will have a tremendous influence in all areas of your life, including school, relationships, careers, leisure time, and health. When managed effectively, stress invites challenge and exhilaration, and motivates you to perform your best. Poorly managed

stress, however, can lead to conflicts in life and to potentially serious health problems.

Since our world is rapidly changing, we need to continually adjust our attitudes and behaviors to keep a state of homeostasis or self-balance. Certain events in our lives will dictate making changes. Being a college student, losing a loved one, and graduating from college are a few examples of transitions in our lives where change is inevitable.

WHAT IS STRESS?

Stress is the rate of wear and tear on the body, including the mind. The word *stress* is used in different ways: as an outside force that causes a person to feel upset or tense, as an internal state of arousal, and as the mental and physical forces that lead to success. Dr. Hans Selye, the father of stress research, defines **stress** as "the nonspecific response of the body to any demand made upon it." In his definition, the body will respond to **stressors** (things that excite us or upset us) similarly, regardless of whether they are a positive or negative event. For example, getting married and being involved in an accident are both stressful. Although one is positive and the other negative, your body cannot tell the two apart, and it will still react the same way.

Distress is negative stress, which can lead to health problems. When it comes to stress, the goal for many people is to have as little as possible. What they may not know is that insufficient stress or stimulation can be as harmful as too much stress, or **distress. Hypostress,** or lack of stimulation, can lead to boredom, loneliness, depression, and, in severe cases, suicide. At the other extreme, too much stress or stimulation (distress) can contribute to heart disease, high blood pressure, indigestion, higher cholesterol levels, low back pain, headaches, ulcers, cancer, and a host of mental disorders.

Eustress is positive stress that contributes to health, high self-esteem, and achievement. Stress can be exhilarating—running a race, getting a promotion, getting a good grade in class, or traveling in a foreign country. This healthy stress is known as **eustress,** or moderate stress. Besides being good stress, eustress is the enhancing stress that overcomes laziness and provides the drive to produce and excel. Each person has a relative stress level that is located somewhere between being too busy and being bored. This comfortable level creates a feeling of well-being that promotes optimal performance and efficiency (see figure 14.1).

The college years can be a time of both positive and negative stress. As a student, you are exposed to a variety of stressors that make your college experience challenging and rewarding. Positive stressors include good grades, satisfying relationships, and achievements in extracurricular activities. Negative stressors include time constraints, such as deadlines, test performance anxiety, noisy and crowded conditions, fear of rejection and failure, career anxiety, fear of the future after schooling, and pressure to conform. Add to this the important decisions that have to be made, such as choosing a major, and you can see why college is a fertile ground for stress (see figure 14.2).

GENERAL ADAPTATION SYNDROME (THE STRESS RESPONSE)

The human body is continually striving to maintain a balanced state known as homeostasis. This

FIGURE 14.1
The Stress Chart

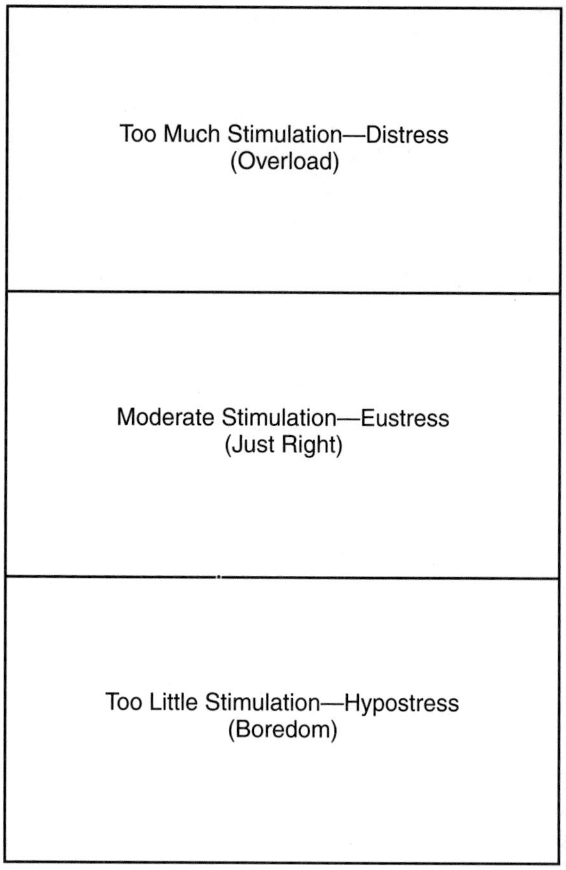

Too Much Stimulation—Distress (Overload)
Moderate Stimulation—Eustress (Just Right)
Too Little Stimulation—Hypostress (Boredom)

FIGURE 14.2
Stressors College Students May Encounter

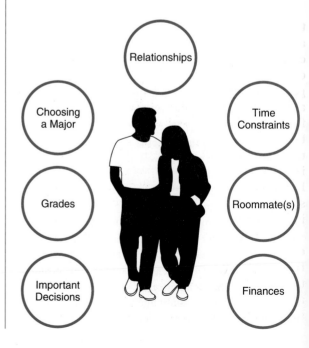

FIGURE 14.3

The Stress Response

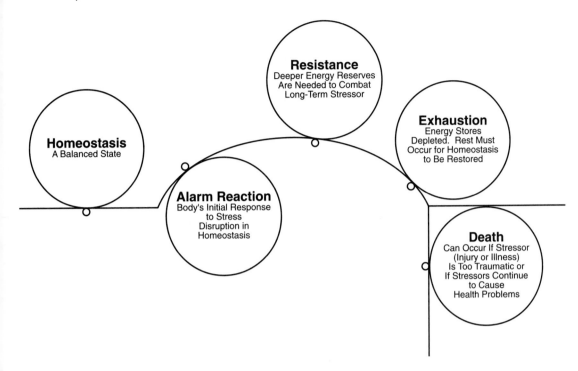

process of adaptation (the stress response) permits an individual to survive a given stressor yet, at the same time, taxes the individual's ability to function. In fact, stress-related diseases such as ulcers and heart disease are termed diseases of adaptation. Many of the diseases that befall us today are chronic or long-term diseases linked to the general adaptation syndrome.

In prehistoric times, our cave-dwelling ancestors were confronted with saber-toothed tigers and other stressors. During those confrontations, a choice had to be made between staying and fighting or running away (**fight or flight**). To survive the dangerous encounters, the cave people's bodies would automatically prepare for action: The heart pumped faster, blood pressure soared, adrenaline poured, blood sugar flowed, muscles tensed, and mental alertness improved. Once the danger was gone, their bodies would return to **homeostasis** (see figure 14.3). Homeostasis is the "internal environment" your body strives to maintain despite wide-ranging differences in the "external environment."

A major change between our cave-dwelling ancestors and us, the people of today, is our ability to think abstractly. The significance of this change is that many of the stressors that we experience today are psychological stressors related to the rapid rate of social change. They are not the physical stressors re-

lated to survival experienced centuries ago. Psychological stressors, like the constant worry about grades, may not have a clear-cut starting point or ending. This, in turn, can lead to their propensity to become chronic sources of stress.

The same stress response encountered by our cave-dwelling ancestors is still with us today and, to some degree, is triggered every time we react to a stressor. What evolved as a self-preserving mechanism can become a health hazard today if the stress is not managed positively.

Being constantly exposed to stressors, whether minor or major, and not managing them well can lead to unwanted health problems. Dr. Selye has identified three stages of the stress response: alarm reaction, resistance, and exhaustion.

Alarm Reaction

The alarm reaction stage is the body's initial response to a stressor being present and homeostasis being disrupted. After the brain perceives a stressor, it automatically prepares the body for fight or flight (see figure 14.4). It does this by triggering mental and physical responses into action. This response is similar to the way our prehistoric ancestors reacted when confronted with danger. Today the stressors are not saber-toothed tigers but deadlines, parental expectations, career anxiety, traffic, negative self-talk, or unhealthy

FIGURE 14.4

How the Body Responds to Stress

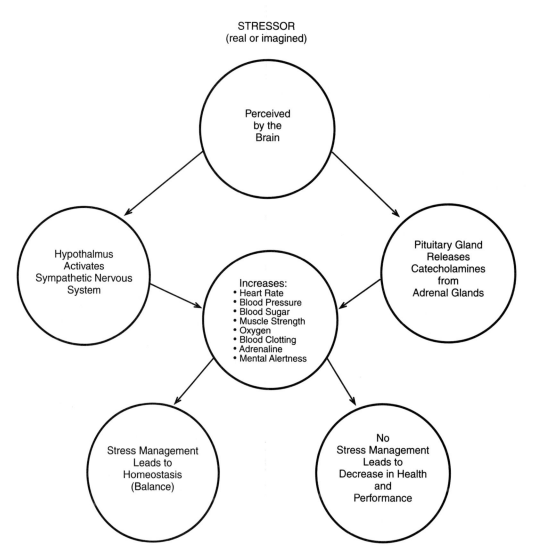

STRESSOR
(real or imagined)

Perceived
by the
Brain

Hypothalmus
Activates
Sympathetic Nervous
System

Increases:
• Heart Rate
• Blood Pressure
• Blood Sugar
• Muscle Strength
• Oxygen
• Blood Clotting
• Adrenaline
• Mental Alertness

Pituitary Gland
Releases
Catecholamines
from
Adrenal Glands

Stress Management
Leads to
Homeostasis
(Balance)

No
Stress Management
Leads to
Decrease in Health
and
Performance

lifestyles. In this first stage, the body responds to the initial stress and usually returns to a balanced state, or homeostasis.

Resistance Stage

The longer our bodies are exposed to the stressor, the greater the opportunity to experience ill effects. In the second stage, known as the resistance stage, the body has advanced beyond the initial response and continues to experience stress. To combat short-term stressors, only superficial levels of energy are required. However, to cope with long-term or intense stressors, the body requires deeper energy reserves.

The use of deeper energy reserves leads to a continued state of unbalance, creating wear and tear within the body. The bottled-up stress that has accu-

mulated from the long-term stressor leaves the person susceptible to mental and physical health problems.

Exhaustion Stage

The exhaustion stage is reached when energy stores have been depleted and rest must occur. The last stage of the stress response is not often reached. Usually, the individual will have successfully removed or coped with the stressor(s) in the alarm and resistance stages. However, if the person has not been able to eliminate or adequately cope with the long-term stressor, exhaustion will occur. If this happens, stress may have already affected the stomach, heart, blood pressure, muscles, joints, and the mind. Death can occur if the stressor (injury or illness) is too traumatic or if the stressor continues to cause health problems. The key to preventing exhaustion and stress-related problems is early intervention through the use of management techniques.

STRESSORS

A stressor is any factor or condition (real or imagined) that initiates the stress response and leads to stress. Stress can be triggered by a wide variety of circumstances, ranging from the death of a loved one to a change in eating and sleeping patterns. The amount of stress you experience will depend on several factors, including your perception of the stressor, the type of stressor, and its intensity and duration.

Categories of Stressors

The three general categories of stressors are cataclysmic, personal, and background. *Cataclysmic stressors* are major catastrophes such as wars and earthquakes that cause tremendous human suffering and great destruction to property. *Personal stressors* such as the loss of a loved one or the breakup of a close relationship are intense in nature and touch individual lives. The most common category consists of *background stressors,* which are persistent, repetitive, daily annoyances (misplacing things, weight concerns, too many things to do) that are part of everyday life.

New events, change, and stress are experienced at every stage of life, from childhood to old age. Just as a seed cannot bear fruit without growth, you cannot mature without stress. With each developmental period of your life and the new changes that accompany it, stress enters your life. Some people are more vulnerable to the stress of life changes than others. Your own personal coping mechanisms will be influenced by many factors. These include your self-concept, past experiences, attitudes toward life, number and frequency of events and changes, and the time and setting in which they occur.

The everyday little hassles (background stressors) may pose more of a health threat than the major life events. Major life events such as divorce and personal injuries are traumatic and can lead to serious health problems. However, they are not the most common enemies to health. It is the everyday minor, frequent annoyances that have the greatest toll on health. Over the days, weeks, and months, the cumulative effect of daily hassles—time constraints, finding a parking place, interruptions, money concerns—becomes more potent than an isolated major event. Your coping strategies to deal with these sometimes unavoidable harassments will largely determine whether you will experience future health problems.

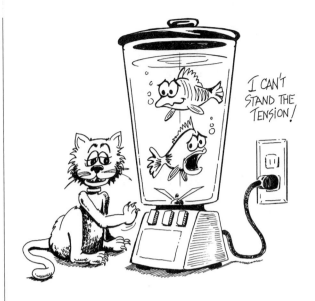

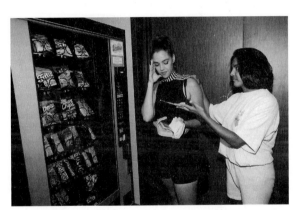

Not having enough money is an example of a negative stressor.

Common Stressors

Psychological, spiritual, physical, social, vocational, and environmental stressors can arise from a variety of situations within a person's everyday life. Psychological stressors are associated with challenging, disturbing, or upsetting thoughts, feelings, and emotions. Spiritual stressors are growth experiences or conflicts in personal, ethical, and moral beliefs. Physical stressors cause us to feel physically challenged (exercise) or uncomfortable (illness). Expectations placed on us by family, friends, and others are social stressors. Vocational stressors are factors or conditions that allow for growth or lead to conflict at the school and work setting. Finally, environmental stressors deal with factors or conditions that affect the planet and, in turn, affect each human being. See figure 14.5 for common stressors that can lead to distress.

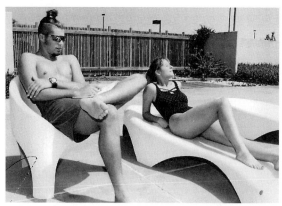

Ultraviolet radiation is a common stressor that can lead to distress.

FIGURE 14.5

Common Stressors That Can Lead to Distress

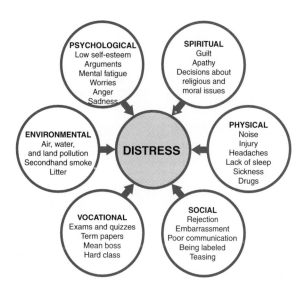

STRESS AND PERSONALITY TRAITS

Types A and B are personality traits that influence the way people cope with stress. A **Type A** personality is typically an overachiever, excessively competitive, impatient, hard driving, high-strung, who may harbor feelings of hostility and anger. Research indicates that a Type A who is always mistrustful, angry, and suspicious is twice as likely to suffer heart disease than other personality types. A **Type B** is usually relaxed, easygoing, and casual, and not prone to serious stress-related illness.

The Hardy personality includes individuals who have a "stress-resistant" style that acts as a buffer against stress. They share three major personality traits known as the three Cs:

- **Commitment:** They have a purpose in life and are committed to family, self, work, and other values.
- **Control:** They exert control over their lives and believe that they can influence their own fate.
- **Challenge:** They see change, and even problems, as a challenge or as opportunities for growth.

The critical factor in how people respond to stress appears to be their level of self-esteem, regardless of personality type. Low self-esteem is the common denominator in stress-prone personalities, and high self-esteem is a prerequisite for building stress-resistant personalities. By placing little or no value on self, we can become vulnerable to our perceptions of stress. Conversely, people with high self-esteem tend to work through their problems and worries without letting negative stress become uncontrollable. Researchers are now strongly advocating ways to raise self-esteem as the primary goal in stress-management programs.

TOLL ON THE BODY

Although stress may be the spice of life, it can also be the kiss of death. Just as stress can stimulate growth, it can also drain mental and physical health. Some medical researchers believe that distress is a primary deterrent to total health and a major contributor to disease. In addition, some medical doctors estimate that as much as 70 percent of all illness may be stress-related.

The mind and body are like teammates—what happens to one affects the other and vice versa. When your mind reacts to a stressor, your body will also respond. When stress is prolonged, it can depress your immune system (the body's army) and lead to a lower resistance to disease. In turn, your body may become host to a multitude of ailments from colds to heart disease (see table 14.1).

BURNOUT

Burnout is a state of psychological and physical exhaustion brought on by constant or repeated demands. Burnout can happen to anyone. Do you usually feel stressed out (unbalanced) at the end of the school term? If so, demands such as term papers and final exams may have overloaded your body's circuits, causing psychological and physical fatigue. You can prevent reaching the end of your rope by being aware of the early warning signs of burnout (see table 14.2) and practicing appropriate coping and relaxation techniques each day.

TABLE 14.1

The Link between Distress and Health

Allergies	Heart disease
Arthritis	High blood pressure
Asthma	Irritable bowel syndrome (stomach pain, bloating, constipation, diarrhea)
Backache	Mental disorders
Cancer	Skin problems
Colds	Strokes
Diabetes	
Hay fever	
Headaches	

TABLE 14.2

Early Warning Signs of Burnout

1. Chronic fatigue
2. Sleep problems or nightmares
3. Increased anxiety or nervousness
4. Muscular tension in the form of headaches, neckaches, shoulderaches, and backaches
5. Increased use of alcohol or medication
6. Digestive problems (nausea, vomiting, or diarrhea)
7. Loss of interest in sex
8. Frequent body aches or pain
9. Quarrels with family or friends
10. A bad attitude about life
11. Problems concentrating; accidents or apathy
12. Feelings of depression, hopelessness, and helplessness

HEALTHY COPING STRATEGIES AND RELAXATION TECHNIQUES

The key to managing stress is to develop healthy coping strategies and practice daily relaxation techniques. The goal in stress management is to maintain balance. Healthy coping strategies and relaxation techniques are effective methods for preventing distress and maintaining eustress. These techniques allow you to turn off harmful bodily effects of stress and counter the negative effects of the fight-or-flight response.

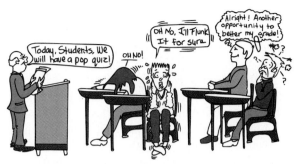

Stressors can be perceived as positive or negative.

HEALTHY COPING STRATEGIES

The use of healthy coping techniques allows you to better deal with the everyday stress of life. Experiment with the different coping techniques to determine which ones work the best for you and incorporate them into your daily routine.

Be in Control

A sense of control may be the single most powerful stress management tool you can use. You have the power to allow or not allow stressors to trigger the stress response. Even though a stressor has been introduced (such as a pop quiz), you can choose to remain calm and in control. From this choice, your body will not experience stress. In this light, you have much more control over yourself and your reactions than you may have previously thought! The key to surviving and thriving in life is to feel in control.

Reframe Your Stressors

Imagine a garden with equal amounts of weeds and flowers. A pessimist will see the garden as half full of weeds, whereas an optimist will see the garden as half full of flowers. Are you mainly a pessimist or an optimist? Reframing is a way of seeing life positively. Most stressors can be perceived in two ways: as a positive challenge or as a negative ordeal. Frequently, it's not the actual event that determines whether you will experience distress or eustress but the "frame" that you put on the stressor.

See Things in Their Proper Perspective

Most of the stressors we experience on a daily basis are relatively minor. However, we frequently allow these minor incidents to become major sources of stress. Why? Because we often fail to view them in their proper perspective. A simple way to remedy this is to ask yourself the following set of questions: How will this incident affect me hours from now? Weeks from now? Months from now? Years from now? By answering these questions, you can more realistically evaluate the significance of the event that is causing stress.

Reduce the Number of Stressors in Your Life

College is a busy time filled with classes, homework, term papers, projects, organizational responsibilities, recreational pursuits, and often a part-time or full-time job. If you are like many college students, you feel "stress overload" from having too many irons in the fire. If you need to, what stressor(s) can you remove to get back into balance?

Be Aware of Early Warning Signs of Distress

Be in tune with your body by recognizing the early warning signs of distress. Some red lights of distress include headaches; tension in the neck, shoulders, and elsewhere; clenched teeth and fists; rapid breathing; rapid heart rate; frustration; and irritability. If you are experiencing these symptoms, practice coping and relaxation techniques.

Early warning signs for lack of stimulation in life include boredom, loneliness, apathy, and a sense of lack of purpose. To help prevent being bored with life, develop a hobby, join an organization, or volunteer your free time to charity.

Enjoy Exercise and Physical Activity

A regular, aerobic exercise program is an excellent strategy for reducing stress. It is a natural way to become relaxed and to renew energy. Exercise reduces the intensity of the stress response, shortens the recovery period from stressful situations, and can even prevent illness in people who are already stressed out. Nervous stomach, headaches, muscle tension, irritability, and aggressiveness disappear or are reduced with exercise.

Be Positive in Your Approach to Life and to Yourself

The relationship you have with yourself is reflected in the relationship you have with the world. By appreciating yourself, you can appreciate the world you live in. You are on the road to high self-esteem if you can magnify your strengths while minimizing your weaknesses. Although most people have doubts and worries from time to time, it is important to replace negative thoughts with positive ones. A heart specialist once said: "Rule 1 is, don't sweat the small stuff; and Rule 2 is, it's all small stuff," and "If you can't fight it and you can't flee—go with the flow."

Worrying can cause headaches, ulcers, and other health-related problems. Be in control of your thoughts by thinking positively and taking action. For

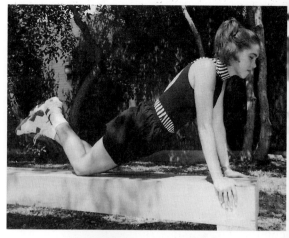

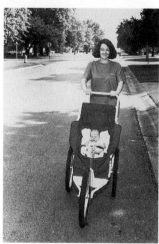

Daily exercise is a healthy way to reduce distress and renew energy.

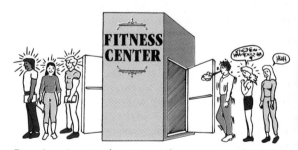

Exercise: A natural way to reduce stress and renew energy.

example, instead of worrying about failing an exam, set yourself up for success by thinking positively about getting a good exam grade. Then follow up by preparing well for the test.

Tap into Your Humor Lifestyle

Warning: Humor may be hazardous to your stress! Laughter and a good sense of humor are powerful stress-reducing agents. Laughter is like aerobic exercise. It relieves muscle tension, head clutter, and makes you feel good all over. Along with laughter, a good sense of humor reinforces positive attitudes and keeps things in perspective by encouraging an appreciation for life (Does life always have to be so serious or predictable?). For lasting health and stress-relieving benefits, medical authorities believe an enduring sense of humor counts more than an occasional laugh.

Strive for Moderation and Balance

Too much of a good thing is wonderful, right? Usually not. Whether it's work, play, sports, exercise, or study, an excess amount of just about anything can lead to distress and health problems. Moderation (a comfortable amount) and balance (being well-rounded) in all areas of life are the keys to happiness and health maintenance.

Use Effective Time Management Skills

How well you spend your time is a critical factor in stress management. Everyone is given twenty-four hours of time each day to spend. It is helpful to prioritize your list of responsibilities on a daily, weekly, monthly, and yearly basis. Write out a list of things that must be done today, this week, this month, and this year. First, accomplish all the tasks that must be done today. The events that are not pending can wait. Routinely adjust your schedule as needed. Keep in mind that successful people spend their time wisely, allowing for a healthy balance among family, school, work, play, and leisure.

Develop Satisfying Relationships

Sharing your life's ups and downs is an important coping strategy for relieving stress and tension. A positive support team consisting of family, friends, and others is a sure way to celebrate life's victories and cope with life's tragedies. Talking, listening, laughing, and crying with your family and close friends do wonders for the heart and mind.

Know When to Ask for Help

In college and throughout life, there may be times when sadness, fear, loneliness, depression, stress, or other problems have control over you. The time to ask for help is when you are not able to work through it by yourself. Family, friends, counselors, physicians, teachers, advisers, ministers, rabbis, and coaches can be helpful during these difficult times.

Abstain from Alcohol or Use Only in Moderation

Drinking alcohol is popular for many college students. Alcohol poses no problem if moderation and good sense are used. This includes knowing when to

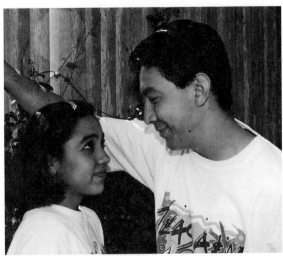

Satisfying relationships can help us work through our problems and cope with life's struggles.

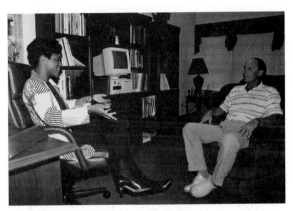

For any psychological problem that becomes unmanageable, or simply for maintenance of the mind, it is important to see a therapist.

stop and not drinking and driving. However, when alcohol is used as an escape from life's problems or is combined with driving, it can actually create more problems. Alcohol-related problems may lead to jail time, fights, unsafe sex, accidents, relationship conflicts, and school failure.

Use Positive Self-Talk

The person you most talk to is yourself. Think about it for a moment. Are your personal conversations mainly positive or negative? When you talk, is there more praise than criticism? Since no one is perfect, there are bound to be wrong decisions and mistakes made in life. Some people get highly upset over spilling a drink or missing one question on an exam. When you find yourself being critical, make a conscious choice to be understanding and see what can be learned from each experience.

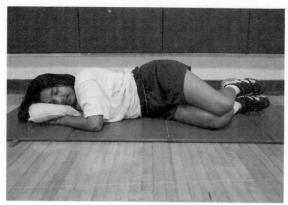

Restful sleep is an important strategy to your stress management program.

Get the Sleep You Need

Most people need six to eight hours of sleep each night. Restful sleep can make you feel alert, calm, patient, and able to handle stress.

Ease Up

Do you have hurry-up-itis? Do you find yourself scurrying from one place to another and from one task to another? This fast-paced lifestyle can take its toll on your body, leaving it susceptible to stress and common ailments. In this busy world, take the time to smell the flowers, hear a bird sing, watch a sunset, and play with a child.

Be Flexible

Life does not always go according to plan. The one thing you can predict accurately in life is that life is unpredictable. Wonderful surprises, terrible tragedies, and many changes await you as you travel on your journey through life. By going with the flow, a flexible person will minimize the stress that usually accompanies the unexpected.

Relaxation Techniques

We can influence our own physical reaction to stress through individually controlled mental practices. Research has found that using relaxation techniques will produce positive physical changes in the body. Some of these healthy changes include feelings of well-being, a lower metabolic rate, lower anxiety levels, and a decrease in heart rate and respiration. Experiment with the relaxation techniques that work best for you. Keep in mind that the long-lasting benefits come to those who practice the techniques regularly.

Quick Relaxation Techniques

When you want instant relief from stress, consider the following suggestions:

1. Inhale deeply and pause for three to five seconds. All at once, let the air out as you relax your jaw and let your shoulders sag. Repeat two to four times.
2. Allow your hips, legs, and feet to relax while sitting in a chair. Visualize them getting heavier and warmer (feelings associated with relaxation).
3. With eyes closed, visualize yourself in an ideal location for relaxation (on a beach, in a cabin, or in your favorite room). Slow down and deepen your breathing as you visually experience the relaxing scene for thirty to sixty seconds.
4. Put your hand on your abdomen. Take a deep breath and exhale, making sure your hand moves up and down. Repeat two to four times.
5. With both hands, gently massage your neck and shoulder muscles.
6. Think of your favorite joke or an amusing though embarrassing moment. If appropriate, laugh until it hurts!

Diversions

To combat the daily hassles of life and for quick relief of stress symptoms, do anything you find relaxing and healthful. Table 14.3 gives some examples of healthy diversions.

Deep Breathing

Deep breathing can be used anywhere and anytime. It can be effectively used before, during, and after a stressful situation (public speaking, taking an exam). To aid in relaxing, you can put on slow tempo music that is flowing, smooth, and calm. The following steps are easy to follow:

1. Lie on the floor in a dimly lit room with your legs and arms extended. If one is available, place a pillow under your knees to take the pressure off your back.
2. Slowly take air into your body through your mouth while extending your abdomen and lower ribs. You want to get oxygen into the lowest part of your lungs.
3. As you repeat, check your lower abdomen for any tension that would inhibit your full, deep breath and allow the tension to release. As you breathe, you should be able to feel the lowest abdominal muscles expand on the intake of air. Your upper chest should not move at all.
4. Let you mind follow the breath in and out of your body, allowing thoughts to simply pass through as you return once again to focusing on your breathing.
5. Sometimes it is helpful to make vocal sounds on the release of the breath. Either the syllable *ah* or

TABLE 14.3
Customized Relaxation Techniques

1. Listen to music.
2. Play with a dog.
3. Enjoy a catnap.
4. Fly a kite.
5. Soak in a bath or hot tub.
6. Chop wood.
7. Call a friend.
8. Listen to a Bill Cosby tape or album.
9. Read.
10. Stargaze.
11. Watch a sunset.
12. Play an instrument.
13. Go fishing.
14. Take in a movie.
15. Play cards.
16. Write in your journal.
17. Volunteer your time.
18. Take a hike.
19. Play a sport.
20. Dance.
21. Listen to a relaxation tape.

TABLE 14.4
Sample Progressive Relaxation Routine

1. Sit up in a chair with the lights dimmed. Remove your shoes and let your feet relax. Arms should also relax in a comfortable position.
2. Once you begin, you'll be proceeding slowly by tensing a muscle group and then relaxing it: Stop if cramping or pain develops.
3. Face: Squint your eyes, wrinkle your nose, make a face, and then relax. Open you mouth very wide, stick out your tongue, clench your teeth, and then relax.
4. Neck: Bring your head downward, touching your chin to your chest. Relax. Try to touch the right ear to right shoulder, and left ear to left shoulder. Relax and center your head.
5. Shoulders: Shrug both shoulders up toward your ears, pull shoulders down from ears, bring shoulders forward, then back. Relax.
6. Hands and Arms: Make a fist. Raise right arm, bending at the elbow and make a muscle with the biceps. Relax. Repeat with left arm. Relax. Bring both arms straight out in front of you. Relax.
7. Back: Bow your back by sticking your abdomen out. Relax. Press lower back into chair. Relax.
8. Abdomen: Suck in abdominal muscles. Relax.
9. Buttocks: Squeeze together buttock muscles. Relax.
10. Thighs: Bring right leg straight out, hold and relax. Do the same for left leg.
11. Calves: Flex toes toward you, then point toes away from your body. Relax.
12. Toes: Curl toes under, first the right foot, then the left foot. Relax.
13. Enjoy for a few moments your state of relaxation.

a word, such as *calm,* can be used. Mentally repeating "I am" on the intake of breath and "relax" on the exhale is also suggested.

6. This exercise can be done for a minute or two or continued for ten to twenty minutes.

Progressive Relaxation

This technique combines the deliberate tensing and relaxing of the muscles. The goal is to identify muscle tension and then relax it. There are many different programs to use in progressive relaxation. You may make up your own or choose a preplanned program (see table 14.4). This form of relaxation is also helpful in treating people with low self-concept, depression, anxiety, and sleep disturbances.

Meditation

Meditation is a simple mental exercise that reduces stress and promotes the relaxation response (see table 14.5). Regardless of cultural sources, two basic elements are important to elicit the relaxation response: (1) the repetition of a word, sound phrase, prayer, image, or physical activity, and (2) a passive disregard of everyday thoughts when they occur during meditation. This concentration helps calm the mind, creating a state of tranquillity. One well-known meditation method was developed by Dr. Herbert Benson of Harvard University. This method involves the steps found in table 14.5.

Autogenic Training and Imagery

In autogenic training, the relaxation response is triggered by using mental exercises to produce sensations of warmth and heaviness in the body. Imagery is added to further the relaxed state by focusing on peaceful scenes. This form of relaxation has been successful in treating individuals with peptic ulcers, high blood pressure, migraine headaches, asthma, and sleep disturbances.

TABLE 14.5

A Sample Program for Meditation

- Sit quietly in comfortable position and close your eyes.

- Deeply relax all your muscles, beginning at the feet and progressing up to the face. Keep them relaxed.

- Breathe easily and naturally through your nose. Become aware of your breathing. As you breathe out, say the word "one" to yourself.

- Continue for 10 to 20 minutes. You may open your eyes to check the time, but do not use an alarm. When you finish, sit quietly for several minutes, at first with your eyes closed and later with your eyes open. Wait several minutes before standing up.

- Do not worry about whether you are successful in achieving a deep level of relaxation. Maintain a passive attitude and permit relaxation to occur at its own pace. When distracting thoughts occur, try to ignore them by not dwelling on them, and return to repeating "one." With practice, the response should come with little effort.

- It is recommended that this be done twice a day, but not within 2 hours after any meal (an active digestive system interferes with meditation).

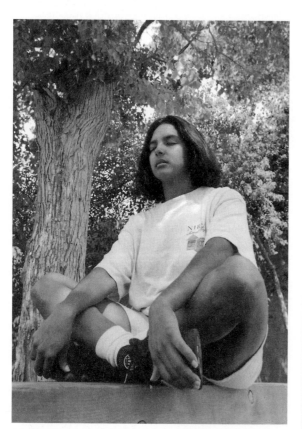

Meditation can reduce stress and promote feelings of well-being.

TABLE 14.6

Steps to Autogenic Training and Imagery Scenes

Autogenic Training

1. Focus on heaviness and warmth of arms and legs, beginning with the dominant side.

2. Focus on warmth and heaviness of heart and chest.

3. Concentrate on breathing rhythm.

4. Concentrate on warmth in the abdominal region.

5. Focus on coolness of forehead.

Imagery Scenes

Sinking into a soft mattress

A soaring bird

Clouds drifting by

A sailboat on a calm lake

Ocean surf splashing on the sand

A feather floating in the sky

Floating in the water

A warm, relaxing fire in the fireplace

A field of pretty flowers

A tree swaying in the wind

After mastering the steps to autogenic training (body relaxation), choose an imagery scene (mental relaxation). You may choose one from table 14.6 or develop your own. To maximize your relaxation, use your senses in the imagery scene. If you are relaxing at the beach, see the blue water, hear the waves pounding the shore, feel the sand between your toes, smell the ocean breeze, and taste the salt from the water.

Biofeedback

Biofeedback training uses machines to measure certain physiological processes. The signals sent back provide biological information such as heart rate, skin temperature, electrical activity of muscles, and blood pressure. From this information, you can learn to control your response to stress. Simple biofeedback methods you can perform on your own include taking your pulse and counting your respiration.

Massage

A favorite technique for relieving muscular tension is massage. Two popular methods are the Swedish massage and shiatsu. Swedish massage involves kneading and rubbing the muscles to improve circulation and increase relaxation. Table 14.7 provides a step-by-step procedure for a shoulder and neck massage.

TABLE 14.7
Should and Neck Massage

1. Have your partner sit straight but comfortably in a chair, relaxed and with eyes closed.

2. From behind, place your hands on your partner's shoulders and begin kneading the two muscles on either side of the neck. Start with very little pressure, then squeeze harder (but not too hard).

3. Next, go to the back of the neck. Position yourself on one side, and have your partner lower his or her head slightly. Support the forehead firmly with one of your hands (this will let your partner's neck muscles relax). With the thumb and first two fingers of your other hand, make tiny circles at the base of the skull.

4. Next, gently squeeze the entire back of the neck and bring your partner's head back to an upright position.

5. Again, position yourself behind your partner. Using the thumb-crawling technique, begin by pressing both thumbs down, one on the outside of each shoulder. Moving them in, press your thumbs firmly at half-inch intervals until both reach the spine at the same time. Now, walk them out again to the shoulders. Repeat this movement several times.

6. Next, with one hand on each shoulder, knead the upper back and shoulders. Work your hands away from one another, ending at the upper arms. Then reverse the process by massaging back to either side of the neck.

7. As a farewell, let your hands come to rest on your partner's shoulders and convey a message of friendship.

Shiatsu, a form of acupuncture, uses pressure applied by the thumbs or fingers to strategic places on the body. The object is to restore balance and have the body's energy flow freely.

Yoga

In yoga, certain postures are combined with rhythmical breathing to remove muscle tension and body stiffness. Yoga performed on a consistent basis can improve mental and physical well-being. To learn yoga, sign up for a class or check out a book.

Flotation Tanks

New on the market are flotation tanks. These devices are soundproof and look like a large bathtub with a shell that closes for complete darkness. Epsom salts are dissolved in warm water for body flotation. This environment eliminates all outside stimuli, creating a sensation of floating in space.

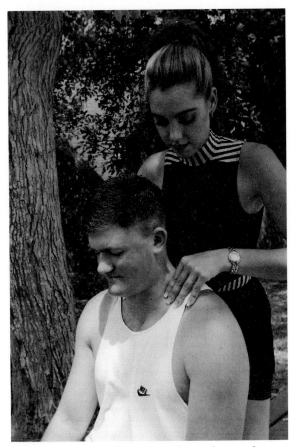

Massage is an excellent relaxation technique for relieving muscular tension.

SUMMARY

- Stress is all around us and is a normal and natural part of life.
- Managed effectively, stress invites challenge and exhilaration and motivates us to perform at our best.
- Managed poorly, stress can lead to conflicts in life and to potentially serious health problems.
- Stress, according to Dr. Hans Selye (father of stress research), is the nonspecific response of the body to any demand placed on it. Whether the stressor is positive (getting married) or negative (accident), the body will react the same.
- Stressors are any factors or conditions that excite us or upset us.
- Distress is defined as an excessive amount of stress. It can contribute to heart disease, high blood pressure, higher cholesterol levels, low back pain, indigestion, headaches, ulcers, cancers, and a host of mental disorders.
- Hypostress is defined as the lack of stimulation. It can lead to boredom, withdrawal, and, in severe cases, suicide.

- Eustress is just the right amount of stress. It contributes to good health, high self-esteem, and achievement.
- The stress response, or how we react to stress, is made up of three stages: (1) alarm reaction (the body's initial response to the stressor); (2) resistance (the body learns to cope with the stressor and begins to use up energy reserves in combating it); and (3) exhaustion (energy stores have been depleted and rest must occur).
- The three general categories of stressors are: cataclysmic (major catastrophes); personal (individual losses); and background (everyday little hassles). The background stressors may pose more of a health threat than cataclysmic or personal stressors because they occur daily.
- Types A and B, and the Hardy personality are personality traits that influence the way people cope with stress. Individuals with a Hardy personality have a "stress-resistant" behavior profile and possess the three Cs: commitment, control, and challenge.
- Prolonged stress often can lead to a host of health problems.
- Burnout is a state of physical and psychological exhaustion that is brought on by constant or repeated demands.
- The key to managing stress is to develop healthy coping strategies and practice daily relaxation techniques.
- Some healthy coping strategies include: be in control, reframe your stressors, reduce the number of stressors in your life, and enjoy exercise and physical activity.
- Some relaxation techniques include diversions, deep breathing, meditation, progressive relaxation, autogenic training and imagery, and massage.

A C T I V I T Y **14A**

LIFE EVENT SCALE FOR THE COLLEGE STUDENT

Name _____ To be submitted: Yes No

Date _____ If yes, due date _____

Class _____ Section _____ Score _____

PURPOSE
1. To determine which of the following events you have experienced within the last year.
2. To measure the likelihood of encountering a stress-related illness.

DIRECTIONS
1. On the Social Readjustment Rating Scale (table 14.8 on page 190) circle the mean value (in column B) associated with all the events you experienced last year.
2. To obtain your score, multiply the number of times an event occurred by its mean value and total your number of points.
3. Check your rating and your implications for illness.

RESULTS
1. What was your score? _____

2. What was your rating? _____

3. What are your chances of suffering from a stress illness or disease within the next year or two? _____

TABLE 14.8

Social Readjustment Rating Scale for College Students

Column A		Life-Change Event	Column B	Column C
_____	(1)	Entered college	50	_____
_____	(2)	Married	77	_____
_____	(3)	Trouble with your boss	38	_____
_____	(4)	Held a job while attending school	43	_____
_____	(5)	Experienced the death of a spouse	87	_____
_____	(6)	Major change in sleep habits	34	_____
_____	(7)	Experienced the death of a close family member	77	_____
_____	(8)	Major change in eating habits	30	_____
_____	(9)	Change in or choice of major field of study	41	_____
_____	(10)	Revision of personal habits	45	_____
_____	(11)	Experienced the death of a close friend	68	_____
_____	(12)	Found guilty of minor violations of the law	22	_____
_____	(13)	Had an outstanding personal achievement	40	_____
_____	(14)	Experienced pregnancy, or fathered a pregnancy	68	_____
_____	(15)	Major change in health or behavior of family member	56	_____
_____	(16)	Had sexual difficulties	58	_____
_____	(17)	Had trouble with in-laws	42	_____
_____	(18)	Major change in number of family get-togethers	26	_____
_____	(19)	Major change in financial state	53	_____
_____	(20)	Gained a new family member	50	_____
_____	(21)	Change in residence or living conditions	42	_____
_____	(22)	Major conflict or change in values	50	_____
_____	(23)	Major change in church activities	36	_____
_____	(24)	Marital reconciliation with your mate	58	_____
_____	(25)	Fired from work	62	_____
_____	(26)	Were divorced	76	_____
_____	(27)	Changed to a different line of work	50	_____
_____	(28)	Major change in number of arguments with spouse	50	_____
_____	(29)	Major change in responsibilities at work	47	_____
_____	(30)	Had your spouse begin or cease work outside the home	41	_____
_____	(31)	Major change in working hours or conditions	42	_____
_____	(32)	Marital separation from mate	74	_____
_____	(33)	Major change in type and/or amount of recreation	37	_____
_____	(34)	Major change in use of drugs	52	_____
_____	(35)	Took on a mortgage or loan of less than $10,000	52	_____
_____	(36)	Major personal injury or illness	65	_____
_____	(37)	Major change in use of alcohol	46	_____
_____	(38)	Major change in social activities	43	_____

TABLE 14.8 (continued)
Social Readjustment Rating Scale for College Students

Column A		Life-Change Event	Column B	Column C
_____	(39)	Major change in amount of participation in school activities	38	_____
_____	(40)	Major change in amount of independence and responsibility	49	_____
_____	(41)	Took a trip or vacation	33	_____
_____	(42)	Engaged to be married	54	_____
_____	(43)	Changed to a new school	50	_____
_____	(44)	Changed dating habits	41	_____
_____	(45)	Trouble with school administration	44	_____
_____	(46)	Broke or had broken a marital engagement or steady relationship	60	_____
_____	(47)	Major change in self-concept or self-awareness	57	_____
			TOTAL	_____

Directions for scoring: List the number of times each event has occurred to you within the past 12 months in Column A. Multiply that by the corresponding numerical value in Column B. Place that number in Column C. Total the scores in Column C.

Interpretation: High Risk 1450 + points

Medium Risk 890 points

Low Risk 347 – points

SOURCE: Martin B. Marx, Thomas F. Garrity, and Frank R. Bowers, "The Influence of Recent Life Experiences on the Health of College Freshmen," Journal of Psychosomatic Research 19 (1975): 97, Copyright 1975, Pergamon Press Ltd.

ACTIVITY *14B*

THE STRESS PROJECT

Name _____   *To be submitted:*   Yes   No

Date _____   *If yes, due date* _____

Class _____   Section _____   Score _____

PURPOSE
To recognize stress in your life and how you managed it.

DIRECTIONS
On the stress log, perform the following:

1. For every hour that you are awake, record any people, situations, or events (stressors) that are stressful to you.

2. For every stressful event, record why it was stressful.

   Try to listen to any self-talk that accompanied your reaction to the stressor. Record what you told yourself that made this a stressor.

3. For each stressful event record how you reacted to the stressor.

4. Answer questions in the Results section.

Stress Log

	Stressors	Why Stressful?	Self-Talk	Reaction to Stressor
Day 1				
Day 2				
Day 3				

	Stressors	Why Stressful?	Self-Talk	Reaction to Stressor
Day 4				
Day 5				
Day 6				
Day 7				

RESULTS

1. During the week of the stress project, which situations or events caused you the most stress?

2. Overall, how do you feel you reacted to your stressors this past week?

3. If you had to do it over again, would you react the same way to your stressors? What changes, if any, would you make the next time?

4. What role did your attitude have on your reactions to your stressors?

5. What stress patterns did you notice during this stress project (i.e., look for recurrent stressors at the same time each day, look for similarities regarding your reaction to various stressors)?

6. Was this stress project worthwhile to you?   Yes   No   In what way(s) could it be improved?

ACTIVITY   *14C*

RELAXATION ACTIVITY

Name _____   **To be submitted: Yes   No**

Date _____   **If yes, due date** _____

Class _____   **Section** _____   **Score** _____

PURPOSE
To acquaint you with several relaxation techniques to determine which ones work the best for stress reduction.

DIRECTIONS
1. Sample at lest three relaxation techniques (deep breathing, progressive relaxation, meditation, autogenic training and imagery, and massage; see pages 184 to 187) in or out of class.

2. You may use the relaxation program outlined in the chapter or make up your own. You may also want to shorten the longer techniques due to time constraints.

RESULTS
1. Which relaxation techniques did you perform?

2. Which ones did you like the most?

3. Do you plan to use any of the relaxation techniques regularly?   Yes   No   If so, which ones?

REFERENCES

American Cancer Society. *Cancer Facts and Figures.* Atlanta, GA: American Cancer Society, 1996.

———. *The Smoke Around You: The Risks of Involuntary Smoking.* Atlanta, GA: American Cancer Society, 1995.

———. *Taking Control: 10 Steps to a Healthier Life and Reduced Cancer Risk.* Atlanta, GA: American Cancer Society, 1992.

American College of Sports Medicine. *Guidelines for Graded Exercise Testing and Exercise Prescription.* 5d ed. Philadelphia: Lea & Febiger, 1995.

———. *The American Heart Association Diet: An Eating Plan for Healthy Americans.* Dallas, TX: American Heart Association, 1993.

———. *1996 Heart and Stroke Facts.* Dallas, TX: American Heart Association, 1995.

American Psychiatric Association. *Diagnostic and Statistical Manual of Mental Disorders.* 3d ed. Washington, DC: American Psychiatric Association, 1987.

Anspaugh, David J., Michael H. Hamrick, and Frank D. Rosato. *Wellness: Concepts and Applications.* 2d ed. St. Louis, MO: Mosby, 1994.

Ardell, Donald B. *The History and Future of Wellness.* Dubuque, IA: Kendall Hunt, 1985.

Ardell, Donald B., and Mark J. Tager. *Planning for Wellness: A Guidebook for Achieving Optimal Health.* 3d ed. Dubuque, IA: Kendall Hunt, 1988.

Bailey, Covert. *The New Fit or Fat.* Boston, MA: Houghton Mifflin, 1991.

Brooks, George A., and Thomas D. Fahey. *Exercise Physiology.* New York: Macmillan, 1985.

———. *Fundamentals of Human Performance.* New York: Macmillan, 1987.

Brown, H. Larry. *Lifetime Fitness.* 3d ed. Scottsdale, AZ: Gorsuch Scarisbrick, 1992.

Callaway, C. Wayne. "Biological Adaptations to Starvation and Semistarvation." In *Obesity and Weight Control,* edited by Reva T. Frankle and Mei-uih Yang, 97–108. Rockville, MD: Aspen Publishers, 1988.

Cheffers, John, and Tom Evaul. *Introduction to Physical Education.* Englewood Cliffs, NJ: Prentice-Hall, 1978.

"Cholesterol: The Villain Revisited." *Nestle Worldview* 4, no. 1 (Spring, 1992). Washington, DC: Nestle Information Service.

Clark, Bruce A. Edited by David K. Leslie. *Mature Stuff: Physical Activity for the Older Adult,* pp. 133–145. Reston, VA: American Alliance for Health, Physical Education, Recreation and Dance, 1989.

Corbin, C., and R. Lindsey. *Concepts of Physical Fitness with Laboratories.* 9th ed. Dubuque, IA: William C. Brown, 1997.

Cox, Frank D. *The AIDS Booklet.* 3d ed. Dubuque, IA: Brown & Benchmark Publishers, 1994.

DeVries, Herbert A. *Physiology of Exercise.* 4th ed. Dubuque, IA: William C. Brown, 1986.

Donatelle, Rebecca J., Lorraine G. Davis, and Carolyn F. Hoover. *Access to Health.* Englewood Cliffs, NJ: Prentice-Hall, 1993.

Feeney, Patricia, ed. *What's in a Label? A Dietitian's Handbook for Helping Consumers Demystify Food Labels.* The American Dietetic Association and ConAgra, Inc., 1990.

"Fifty Simple Ways to Improve Your Diet." *Tufts University Diet and Nutrition Letter* 10, no. 4 (June 1992).

Fisher, S. *Stress and Perception of Control.* Hillsdale, NJ: Lawrence Erlbaum, 1984.

FLI Learning Systems. *The Big Click: Safety Belts.* Princeton, NJ: FLI Learning Systems, 1985.

Fox, Edward L., and Richard W. Bowers. *Sports Physiology.* 3d ed. Dubuque, IA: William C. Brown, 1992.

Fox, Edward L., Richard W. Bowers, and Merle L. Foss. *The Physiological Basis for Physical Education and Athletics.* 4th ed. Dubuque, IA: William C. Brown, 1989.

Friedman, Rodney M., ed. "Fatter Calories." *University of California at Berkeley Wellness Letter* 5 (October 1988): 1–2.

Getchell, Bud. *Physical Fitness, A Way of Life.* 4th ed. New York: Macmillan, 1992.

Giordano, Daniel A., and George S. Everly, Jr. *Controlling Stress and Tension: A Holistic Approach.* 2d ed. Englewood Cliffs, NJ: Prentice-Hall, 1986.

"Global AIDS Experts Paint Grim Picture." Jackson (Miss.) *Clarion Ledger,* 19 July 1992.

"Government Gives New Shape to Eating Right." *Tufts University Diet and Nutrition Letter* 10, no. 5 (July 1992).

Greenberg, Jerrold S. *Comprehensive Stress Management.* 2d ed. Dubuque, IA: William C. Brown, 1987.

Greenberg, Jerrold S., and David Pargman. *Physical Fitness: A Wellness Approach.* 2d ed. Englewood Cliffs: NJ: Prentice-Hall, 1989.

Griffith, R. O., R. H. Dressendorfer, C. D. Fullbright, and C. E. Wade, "Testicular Function During Exhaustive Endurance Training." *The Physician and Sportsmedicine* 18, no. 5 (1990): 54, 56.

Hales, Dianne. *An Invitation to Health.* 7th ed. Redwood City, CA: Benjamin/Cummings, 1997.

Hamrick, Michael H., David J. Anspaugh, and Gene Ezell. *Health.* Columbus, OH: Charles E. Merrill, 1986.

Hawkins, Jerald D., and Sandra M. Weigle. *Walking for Fun and Fitness.* Englewood, CO: Morton Publishing, 1992.

Hesson, James L. *Weight Training for Life.* 3d ed. Englewood, CO: Morton Publishing, 1995.

Hockey, Robert V. *Physical Fitness: The Pathway to Healthful Living.* St. Louis, MO: Times Mirror/Mosby College Publishing, 1989.

InfoMatters, American Council on Exercise. "Monitoring Exercise Intensity Using Heart Rate." Vol. 1., no. 1., Sept./Oct. 1995.

Insel, Paul M., and Walton T. Roth. *Concepts in Health.* 7th ed. Mountain View, CA: Mayfied, 1994.

Johnson, Barry L., and Jack K. Nelson. *Practical Measurements for Evaluation in Physical Education.* New York: Macmillan, 1986.

Kanner, Allen, James Coyne, Catherine Schaefer, and Richard Lazarus. "Comparison of Two Modes of Stress Management: Daily Hassles and Uplifts Versus Major Life Events." *Journal of Behavior Medicine* 4, no. 1 (January 1981).

Katch, Frank I., and William D. McArdle. *Nutrition, Weight Control and Exercise.* 2d ed. Philadelphia: Lea and Febiger, 1983.

Keesey, Richard E. "A Set-Point Theory of Obesity." In *Handbook of Eating Disorders,* edited by Kelly D. Brownell and John P. Foreyt, 63–87. New York: Basic Books, 1986.

Kemper, D. K., J. Giuffre, and G. Drabinski. *Pathways: A Successful Guide for a Healthy Life.* Boise, ID: Healthwise, Inc., 1985.

"Key Aspects of the New Nutritional Label." *FDA Consumer.* Vol. 23. May, 1993.

Kusinitz, Ivan, and Morton Fine. *Your Guide to Getting Fit.* 2d ed. Mountain View, CA: Mayfield, 1991.

Lamb, David R. *Physiology of Exercise.* 2d ed. New York: Macmillan, 1984.

Levy, Marvin R., Mark Dignan, and Janet H. Shirreffs. *Life and Health: Targeting Wellness.* New York: McGraw-Hill, 1992.

Luckman, Joan. *Your Health.* Englewood Cliffs, NJ: Prentice-Hall, 1990.

Luttgens, Kathryn, and Katharine F. Wells. *Kinesiology.* 7th ed. Dubuque, IA: William C. Brown, 1989.

"Maintaining a Healthy Weight." *Nestle Worldview* 4, no. 1 (Spring, 1992). Washington, DC: Nestle Information Service.

Mathis, Deborah. "Without Information, Onslaught of Adolescent AIDS Cases May Occur." Jackson (Miss.) *Clarion Ledger,* 28 July 1992.

Mayer, Jean. *A Diet for Living.* New York: David McKay Co., 1975.

———. "An Hour of Exercise vs. a Pound of Flesh." In *Overweight and Obesity: Causes, Fallacies, Treatment,* edited by Brent Q. Hafen, 343–345. Provo, UT: Brigham Young University Press, 1975.

McArdle, William D., Frank I. Katch, and Victor L. Katch. *Exercise Physiology.* 3d ed. Philadelphia: Lea & Febiger, 1991.

McGlynn, George. *Dynamics of Fitness: A Practical Approach.* 4th ed. Dubuque, IA: William C. Brown, 1996.

Miller, David K., and T. Earl Allen. *Fitness, A Lifetime Commitment.* 4th ed. New York: Macmillan, 1990.

Morrison's Custom Management. *Nutrition Choices for a Healthful Lifestyle.* Mobile, AL: Morrison's Custom Management, 1992.

Morrison's Custom Management. *Strides for Life Walking and Nutrition Education Program.* Mobile, AL: Morrison's Custom Management, 1992.

"The New Food Labels." *University of California at Berkeley Wellness Letter,* vol. 9, March, 1993.

Piscopo, John. *Fitness and Aging.* New York: John Wiley and Sons, 1985.

Powers, Scott K., and Edward T. Howley. *Exercise Physiology.* Dubuque, IA: William C. Brown, 1990.

Prentice, William E. *Get Fit, Stay Fit.* St. Louis, MO: Mosby Year Book, 1996.

———. *Fitness for College and Life.* 3d ed. St. Louis, MO: Mosby Year Book, 1991.

Research Matters, American Council on Exercise. *Healthy People 2000: Are We Halfway There Yet?* Vol. 1., no. 3., Sept./Oct. 1995.

Robbins, Gwen, Debbie Powers, and Sharon Burgess. *A Wellness Way of Life.* 2d ed. Dubuque, IA: William C. Brown, 1994.

Seiger, Lon, and James Hesson. *Walking for Fitness.* 3d ed. Dubuque, IA: William C. Brown, 1997.

Seiger, Lon, and Jan Richter. *Your Health, Your Style: Strategies for Wellness.* Dubuque, IA: William C. Brown, 1997.

Selye, Hans. *Stress without Distress.* New York: J. B. Lippincott, 1984.

Sherman, R. "The Big Push, Federal Prosecutors Pump Iron into Their Campaign Against Bodybuilding Steroids." *The National Law Journal* 14, no. 23 (1992): 40.

Siedentop, Daryl. *Introduction to Physical Education, Fitness, & Sport.* Mountain View, CA: Mayfield, 1990.

Siegel, Arthur J. "New Insights about Obesity and Exercise." *Your Patient and Fitness* 2, no. 6 (Nov./Dec., 1988).

Silvester, L. Jay. *Weight Training for Strength & Fitness.* Boston, MA: Jones & Bartlett, 1992.

Steinmetz, J., J. Blankenship, L. Brown, D. Hall, and G. Miller. *Managing Stress Before It Manages You.* Palo Alto, CA: Bull Publishing, 1980.

Surgeon General's Report on Physical Activity and Cardiovascular Health. Washington, D.C., July 11, 1996.

Taste Matters, American Council of Exercise. *Folic Acid: Not Just For Pregnant Women Anymore.* Vol. 2. no. 1., January/February 1996.

Tortora, Gerard J., & Nicholas P. Anagnostakos. *Principles of Anatomy & Physiology.* New York: Harper & Row, 1990.

Turner, L. W., F. S. Sizer, E. N. Whitney, and B. B. Wilks. *Life Choices: Health Concepts and Strategies.* 2d ed. St. Paul, MN: West, 1992.

U.S. Department of Agriculture, U.S. Department of Health and Human Resources. *Nutrition and Your Health: Dietary Guidelines for Americans.* 4th ed. Washington, DC: Government Printing Office, 1996.

Van Itallie, Theodore B., and John G. Kral. "The Dilemma of Morbid Obesity." *Journal of the American Medical Association* 246 (August 28, 1981): 999–1003.

"Vitamins: Building Blocks of Better Health." *Nestle Worldview* 3, no. 4 (Winter, 1992). Washington, DC: Nestle Information Service.

"Weighing the Facts on Obesity." *Nestle Worldview* 4, no. 1 (Spring, 1992). Washington, DC: Nestle Information Service.

Wellness Guide for Older Adults. Marketing Services, Pennsylvania Hospital, Philadelphia, PA: 19107–6192, p. 12.

Wilmore, Jack H., and David L. Costil. *Training for Sport and Activity.* 3d ed. Dubuque, IA: William C. Brown, 1988.

INDEX